An Introduction to Medical Teaching

William B. Jeffries · Kathryn N. Huggett
Editors

An Introduction to Medical Teaching

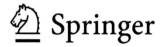 Springer

Editors
Dr. William B. Jeffries
University of Vermont
College of Medicine
Office of Medical Education
Burlington VT 05405
E-125 Given Bldg.
USA
William.B.Jeffries@med.uvm.edu

Dr. Kathryn N. Huggett
Creighton University
School of Medicine
2500 California Plaza
Omaha NE 68178
USA
KathrynHuggett@creighton.edu

ISBN 978-90-481-3640-7   e-ISBN 978-90-481-3641-4
DOI 10.1007/978-90-481-3641-4
Springer Dordrecht Heidelberg London New York

Library of Congress Control Number: 2009943719

Printed on acid-free paper

Springer is part of Springer Science+Business Media (www.springer.com)

Preface

This book was conceived as a tool for the many varieties of medical teacher: the basic scientist, the clinical faculty member, the resident physician and the community practitioner. Individuals from each of these groups often assume the responsibility for educating the physicians of tomorrow. However, the formal training of these teachers is usually not centered on educational principles. Medical teachers often enter their careers ill equipped to engage in a scholarly approach to teaching. Thus we chose to create this volume as a how-to guide for medical teachers who wish to gain an understanding of educational principles and apply them to their teaching.

In keeping with the spirit of the book as an introduction, we have not produced a comprehensive textbook on medical education. Rather, the book is intended to introduce the reader to a variety of major topics that might serve specific needs. This work will be particularly useful to the educator who wants to introduce new methods into their teaching. As such, all of the chapters are grounded in the modern literature underlying adult learning theory and educational methods; however, the advice contained in each chapter is overwhelmingly practical and can be put to immediate use. The chapters begin with a focus on the learner, followed by a survey of the most common teaching modalities encountered by a medical teacher (large group, small group, problem-based, team based, clinical, simulation, and laboratory). We also examine critical elements that comprise the essentials of teaching and learning (using technology, student assessment, teaching evaluation, course design). Finally, we introduce the topic of educational scholarship and supply advice on documenting teaching for career advancement. In addition, to encourage the reader to further investigate each topic, chapters are fully referenced and the appendix provides additional educational resources.

The scope of educational scholarship is now quite broad. Thus no single author could adequately address the topics presented herein. We have thus assembled an exceptionally qualified and highly regarded team of authors who represent a diverse pool of teachers, clinicians and educational scholars. We are extremely grateful to the authors, who generously devoted their time and talents to this project.

Contents

Contributors

Mark A. Albanese, PhD University of Wisconsin School of Medicine and Public Health, Madison, WI, USA

M. Brownell Anderson, MEd Association of American Medical Colleges, Washington, DC, USA

Karen J. Brasel, MD, MPH Medical College of Wisconsin, Milwaukee, WI, USA

David A. Cook, MD, MHPE Mayo Clinic College of Medicine, Rochester, MN, USA

Kristi J. Ferguson, PhD University of Iowa Carver College of Medicine, Iowa City, IA, USA

Kathryn N. Huggett, PhD Creighton University School of Medicine, Omaha, NE, USA

William B. Jeffries, PhD University of Vermont College of Medicine, Burlington, VT, USA

Brian Mavis, PhD College of Human Medicine, Michigan State University, East Lansing, MI, USA

Kathryn K. McMahon, PhD Department of Medical Education, Paul L. Foster School of Medicine, Texas Tech University Health Sciences Center, El Paso, TX, USA

Susan J. Pasquale, PhD University of Massachusetts Medical School, Worcester, MA, USA

Christopher B. Reznich, PhD College of Human Medicine, Michigan State University, East Lansing, MI, USA

Janet M. Riddle, MD, FACP Department of Medical Education, University of Illinois-Chicago, College of Medicine, Chicago, IL, USA

Nicole K. Roberts, PhD Southern Illinois University School of Medicine, Springfield, IL, USA

Deborah Simpson, PhD Medical College of Wisconsin, Milwaukee, WI, USA

Carole S. Vetter, MD Medical College of Wisconsin, Milwaukee, WI, USA

Travis P. Webb, MD Medical College of Wisconsin, Milwaukee, WI, USA

Chapter 1
Facilitating Student Learning

Kristi J. Ferguson

Helping students learn in medical education presents unique challenges that have changed rapidly over the last 10 years. For example, the growth of medical knowledge is accelerating exponentially, making it impossible for prospective physicians to learn everything they need to know during medical school, and making it essential for them to learn the skills related to lifelong learning that will serve them for their entire medical careers. Prospective physicians must learn how to identify their own learning needs, identify appropriate sources for addressing those needs, and learn how to apply the information and skills acquired to the care of patients during medical school and beyond. In addition, traditional models that feature pre-clinical training followed by 2 years of clinical training are giving way to newer models, which emphasize early application of basic science knowledge to clinical problems (e.g., through problem-based learning), as well as revisiting basic science content in the clinical years.

While growth in knowledge creates the need for lifelong learning, characteristics of students and their access to technology have changed as well. For example, incoming students have grown up with access to technology, and are accustomed to using it in their daily lives. This creates advantages as well as challenges for the medical educator. Using technology to store information for later retrieval is easy; being critical of available information and identifying sources of information that are valid is more difficult. Newer high-fidelity simulation allows students to learn and practice skills before they use them on patients, it provides opportunities for learning to work in teams to solve critical problems without putting patients at risk, and it provides a mechanism for assessing these skills in an authentic setting.

Later chapters in this book will address specific educational methods, e.g., Chapter 2 looks at the use of large group teaching methods, Chapter 3 addresses the use of small groups, Chapter 4 looks at problem-based learning, and Chapter 7 looks at simulation. Others will address issues of concern to the field in general, such as assessment of students, evaluation of teaching and learning, scholarship, and planning.

K.J. Ferguson (✉)
University of Iowa Carver College of Medicine, Iowa City, IA, USA

W.B. Jeffries, K.N. Huggett (eds.), *An Introduction to Medical Teaching*,
DOI 10.1007/978-90-481-3641-4_1, © Springer Science+Business Media B.V. 2010

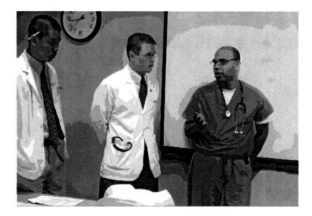

This chapter will begin with a discussion of key concepts related to helping students learn. It will then cover student-centered approaches, such as self-directed learning, that can enhance learning with understanding. Next, it will review the role of the teacher in developing appropriate learning activities and assessment strategies, and will conclude with a discussion of the role of feedback and the learning environment in enhancing student learning.

Key Terms

Active learning refers to instructional approaches that require learners to interact with the material in some fashion, as opposed to being passive recipients of information.

Self-directed learning means that learners control the objectives as well as the approach to their learning. It can also refer to control over the methods used to assess learning. Self-directed learning is more a matter of degree than an all-or-nothing proposition.

Surface learning refers to acquiring knowledge through memorization, without reflecting on it, and the main purpose of surface learning is often to meet external requirements.

Deep learning, on the other hand, relates prior knowledge to new information, integrates information across courses, and organizes content into a coherent knowledge base. Motivation for deep learning is more internal (to the student).

Scaffolding refers to assistance that students receive early on in their learning that is gradually taken away as students become more responsible for their own learning.

Learning environment in this chapter refers to the extent to which the overall organization of learning and support services demonstrates concern for students' well-being as well as for their academic achievement. The **hidden curriculum** refers to learning that occurs outside the classroom, and in medical education often refers to behavior observed by learners that demonstrates such attributes as honesty, respect, and professional values (or their absence).

Role of Learners

Marchese (1998) discusses several criteria that are associated with long-term learning and retention (see Table 1.1). Independent learning, having choices about what to learn, and building on students' intrinsic motivation and natural curiosity all present special challenges for medical educators. External forces such as accrediting bodies and licensing boards have a significant impact on the context of what medical students have to learn. Even so, it is possible to build more self-directed, motivating ways of learning into the curriculum. For example, one of the major benefits of problem-based learning is that students enjoy learning and spend more of their time in independent, self-directed learning. Team-based learning, which builds small group learning activities into large classes, may offer some of the benefits of problem-based learning within a more traditional structure. In addition, hybrid curricula that incorporate self-directed, small group learning experiences alongside traditional classes may offer some of the benefits of problem-based learning while maintaining some of the efficiency of large group teaching.

Table 1.1 Criteria associated with long-term learning and retention (Adapted from Marchese, 1998)

Role of the learner
- Learners function independently
- Learners have choices about what to learn and how to learn
- Learners have opportunities to build on intrinsic motivation and natural curiosity

Role of the learning activities
- Learning activities require the application of higher-order thinking skills
- Learning activities mirror the tasks that learners will face in the real world

Role of feedback and assessment
- Learners are able to practice and receive feedback in challenging interactions with other learners, with minimal threat
- Learners receive frequent feedback and are encouraged to reflect on the feedback
- Learners are assessed in ways that mirror the above criteria

No matter what strategy is used, it is important to maintain students' natural curiosity about how the human body works and about how to take care of patients. Most students come to medical school with high levels of curiosity, but the more they are required to memorize isolated facts or engage in very deep learning about relatively esoteric principles, the less likely they are to maintain that enthusiasm. The challenge comes in identifying core material and teaching it in an interesting, clinically relevant manner.

Another aspect of the role of the learner concerns individual learning style. While learning style has been studied extensively, claims have been made based on minimal evidence in terms of the effect of learning style on learning outcomes, or of designing instruction to match an individual's learning style. That being said, there is little harm in designing instruction that has the potential to meet the needs of students with varying learning styles. A traditional method to reinforce material in multiple ways is to offer instruction that students can both see and hear. For example, a lecture with slides and accompanying written materials reinforces the material in multiple ways. Other variants of learning style indicate whether the learner prefers to learn alone or with others. Since medical practice often involves interacting with other professionals as well as with patients, having practice interacting with colleagues in a learning environment is important even if an individual student's general preference is to work alone.

Role of the Teacher

How students learn is affected by how teachers teach. A model presented by Kern et al. (1998) and others is especially helpful in looking at the process of developing curriculum in medical education (see Fig. 1.1). Kern and colleagues talk about the importance of first doing a needs assessment, to determine what learners already know and what they need to know. Then the teacher must develop goals and objectives for learners. Once this process is complete, educators must develop strategies that will be effective in reaching those goals and objectives. Finally, the teacher must assess learners in ways that reflect the goals, objectives, and strategies.

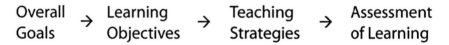

Fig. 1.1 Aligning goals, objectives, strategies, and assessment

Writing Objectives, Developing Strategies, and Designing Assessment Plans

In medical education, decisions about curriculum content are often made without first determining the overall goals and learning objectives. Goals are statements about the overall purposes of a curriculum. Objectives must be specific and measurable, and can be related to the learner, the process, or the outcomes of education. Each must be written in a way that allows for measurement to determine whether the objective has been achieved. Then strategies must be selected that allow the learner to achieve the desired objectives. Once the curriculum has been implemented, learners and the curriculum are evaluated, feedback is provided, and the cycle continues. Too often, educators select a teaching strategy without a clear idea of what they are trying to accomplish, e.g., incorporating small group teaching methods without understanding what such methods can reasonably accomplish or when they can be used most effectively.

Kern et al., discuss five types of objectives, each of which is most appropriately addressed by different types of educational strategies. For example, cognitive objectives related to knowledge acquisition can be taught by readings and lectures, while problem solving can be learned through problem-solving exercises or learning

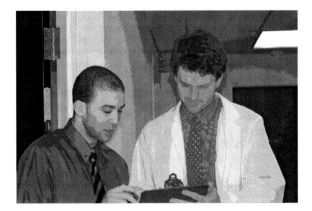

projects. Affective objectives may be achieved most appropriately through discussion, psychomotor skills must be demonstrated and practiced, while behavioral objectives may require real life experiences to be achieved.

Role of Learning Activities

Learning with understanding, as described in "How People Learn" (2000), assumes that a strong knowledge base of facts is important, but not sufficient for learning. Knowledge must be organized around important concepts, which improves understanding and ability to apply the knowledge to other contexts. Obtaining a large knowledge base involves being exposed to multiple examples of a given concept, active processing of the information, and use of higher-order thinking skills in working with the facts. Bloom's Taxonomy has been cited widely in educational circles. An approach that may be even more useful in medical education is Quellmalz' Taxonomy (see Table 1.2). The five levels are **Recall, Analysis, Comparison, Inference** and **Evaluation.**

At the **Recall** level, students remember key facts, and are asked to repeat them, either verbatim or by paraphrase. At the **Analysis** level, students break down a concept into separate components, and may look at cause/effect relationships. At the **Comparison** level, students are required to explain similarities and differences. At the **Inference** level, students may be given a generalization and asked to explain it, or they may be given the evidence and be asked to come up with a generalization. At the **Evaluation** level, students are asked to judge the worth of a particular statement or idea.

In order to encourage higher-order thinking, the goal should be to identify objectives, design teaching strategies, and assess learners at levels that are deeper than simple recall of information. While learners need to have certain basic facts, it is in analyzing, comparing, drawing inferences, and evaluating information that learning for understanding occurs.

Table 1.2 Taxonomy of thinking skills (Adapted from Stiggins et al., 1988)

Category	Description	Sample questions and tasks
Recall	• Remembering or recognizing key facts, definitions, concepts. • Repeating verbatim or paraphrasing information that has already been provided to the student.	• Define the word digestion. • List the vital signs. • What is a normal blood pressure? • Name the amino acids.
Analysis	• Understanding relationships between the whole and its component parts and between cause and effect. • Sorting and categorizing. • Understanding how things work and how the parts of something fit together. • Understanding causal relationships. • Getting information from charts, graphs, diagrams, and maps. • Reflectively structuring knowledge in new ways.	• In what sequence did the symptoms occur? • How does a blood pressure cuff work? • Use the values provided to determine whether the patient is acidotic.
Comparison	• Explaining how things are similar and how they are different. • Comparisons may be either simple or complex. • Simple comparisons are based on a small number of very obvious attributes. • Complex comparisons require an examination of a more sensitive set of attributes of two or more things. • Comparisons start with the whole/part relationships in the analysis category and carry them a step further.	• In what ways are pneumonia and asthma alike? In what ways do they differ? • Compare the risks and benefits to treatment of these.
Inference	• Reasoning inductively or deductively. • In deductive tasks, students reason from generalizations to specific instances and are asked to recognize or explain the evidence. • In inductive tasks, students are given the evidence or details and are required to relate and integrate the information to come up with the generalization.	• What would happen if the patient lost 30 pounds? • Predict what will be the result if you stopped the patient's blood pressure medication. • Based on your research, what can you conclude about the need for this biopsy?
Evaluation	• Expressing and defending an opinion. • Evaluation tasks require students to judge quality, credibility, worth, or practicality using established criteria and explain how the criteria area met or not met.	• Is the experiment designed so that you will be able to tell whether the treatment is more effective than placebo? • What is the most cost-effective way to diagnose pulmonary embolisms?

Requiring students to apply and integrate material may also require faculty members and course directors to integrate material across courses as well as across years of the curriculum. This means that faculty members need to know what is being taught in other courses, and, as much as possible, to reinforce learning that is going on in other courses. In a hybrid curriculum, this would mean that cases for problem-based learning sessions are identified and selected based on the cases' ability to provide clinical relevance for what is being learned in the basic sciences, and for integrating material across courses.

Role of Feedback and Assessment

Another criterion identified by Marchese (1998) i.e., giving learners frequent feedback and encouraging them to reflect on the feedback, can be challenging in medical education as well. For example, evidence about the accuracy of learners' self-assessment suggests that higher achieving students tend to underestimate their performance while lower achieving students tend to over-estimate their performance. This makes the role of feedback and mentoring especially critical in helping students improve.

In the pre-clinical curriculum, too often the only form of feedback is exam scores, and there is often not enough time for students to reflect on exam performance and learn from their mistakes. The focus for reflecting on individual and class performance should be to identify areas of misunderstanding, and to identify ways in which the teaching or preparing for exams can be improved. Methods of assessment and feedback have powerful effects on student motivation. Giving students multiple chances for practice and feedback, for everything from interviewing skills and professional communication to knowledge about anatomy, can go a long way toward enhancing student learning. Doing so with groups of learners, so they can learn from each other, can be especially valuable, as long as the opportunities for practice and feedback occur in an environment supportive of learning and of the students. The key is to be sure that the assessment methods reward higher-order thinking skills.

Following are examples of general goals, learning objectives related to the goals, learning strategies appropriate for achieving the objectives, and methods for evaluating both learners and the process to determine whether goals and objectives have been achieved. Let's consider a hypothetical course entitled "Foundations of Clinical Practice."

One overall goal for Foundations of Clinical Practice is for the student to become a competent, compassionate, and ethical clinician. An objective related to that goal is for the student to develop basic skills in conducting and summarizing the patient interview. Strategies for helping students achieve this goal include lectures, small group discussion and practice, and interaction with simulated patients. Lectures address general communication skills, specific components of taking a history, and dealing with patients' emotions. Small group sessions provide students with multiple opportunities to practice these skills before they interact with simulated patients. Assessment strategies include evaluations by the simulated patients, written exam

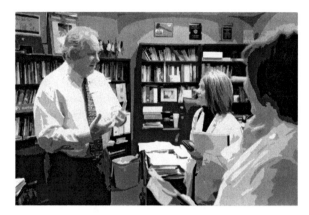

questions related to factual knowledge about elements of the history, and essay questions that require students to demonstrate that they know what questions to ask to
characterize a symptom for a written case scenario.

Another example of an overall goal is to teach students to apply relevant basic
and clinical science principles to the practice of medicine. One objective states
that the course will help students integrate information learned in other courses in
a clinically meaningful way. This is accomplished primarily through small group
discussion in problem-based learning groups. Assessment includes facilitator evaluations, peer evaluations, written tests over the terminology, and a one-page essay
question that asks students to write as though they were talking to the patient in the
problem-based learning case in order to explain the diagnosis, explain what is caus-
ing the problem, describe how the lab tests and history confirmed the diagnosis, and
tell the patient what to expect from the treatment.

The Learning Environment

How well students learn is influenced by a variety of factors. Their own prior
knowledge and motivation are certainly important. Input from their fellow students,
especially if instruction is designed to take advantage of collaborative learning, can
also be important. The environment can also have a profound effect on learning.
For example, is the physical environment arranged so that students have easy access
to study space? Is the schedule organized to maximize student learning? Are services such as tutoring or study groups available for students who need them? Does
the learning environment in the preclinical years minimize unnecessary competition? Do faculty members set realistic standards for what students are expected to
achieve? During the clinical years, do faculty members and residents serve as role
models in the compassionate and ethical treatment of patients? Do they demonstrate professionalism in interactions with colleagues? Creating a collaborative
learning environment is particularly challenging in medical education, as students
who are admitted to medical school often have gotten there because of individual

achievement, not because they have been working in collaborative learning environments. Yet medicine is not practiced in isolation. Physicians must know how to work with other professionals and with their patients. So it is important to create a learning environment in which collaboration is encouraged.

Take Home Points

- Exponential growth in medical knowledge requires new approaches in medical education.
- Long-term retention of knowledge requires active processing of information and use of higher-order thinking skills.
- Students who have choices about their learning and can maintain intrinsic motivation will learn better and be able to apply their knowledge outside the classroom.
- Teachers have an important role in designing learning activities and assessment strategies that foster independent learning and higher-order thinking skills.
- Frequent feedback and reflection are important components in self-directed learning.
- Working in a supportive learning environment that reinforces self-directed learning and professional behavior can enhance student learning.

References

Commission on Behavioral and Social Sciences and Education, National Research Council (2000) How people learn. In: Brain, mind, experience, and school. National Academy Press, Washington, DC, Available via http://www.nap.edu

Kern DE, Thomas PA, Howard DM, Bass EB (1998) Curriculum development for medical education: A six-step approach. Johns Hopkins University Press, Baltimore, MD.

Marchese TJ (1998) The new conversations about learning insights from neuroscience and anthropology, cognitive science and workplace studies. In: New horizons for learning. Available via http://www.newhorizons.org/lifelong/higher_ed/marchese.htm

Stiggins RJ, Rubel E, Quellmalz E (1988) Measuring thinking skills in the classroom, rev ed. National Education Assn Professional Library, West Haven, CT.

For Further Reading

Ferguson KJ (2005) Problem-based learning: Let's not throw the baby out with the bathwater. Medical Education Apr 39(4): 352–353.

This is an editorial responding to criticism of problem-based learning.

Team Based Learning Collaborative, Website: http://www.tlcollaborative.org/

This website is a great resource for those interested in learning more about team-based learning.

Eva KW, Regehr G (2005) Self-assessment in the health professions: A reformulation and research agenda. Academic Medicine 2 Oct 80(10): S46–S54.

This article reviews the evidence related to self-assessment, and recommends approaches for improving self-assessment.

Chapter 2
Teaching Large Groups

William B. Jeffries

Despite many innovations in teaching and learning methods, the 1 hour lecture remains a mainstay of medical education. For many faculty, the lecture is seen as an irreplaceable way to inform students about essential aspects of important subjects. However, for some the lecture format conjures up visions of students sitting long hours in their seats, passively listening to an expert expound on an esoteric topic. A large body of educational research has cast doubt on the amount of learning that actually takes place during a traditional lecture. The data show that while this format can be an effective way to transfer knowledge to students, it is not more effective than other methods (Bligh, 2000). Further, the lecture is usually not the most optimal way to teach skills or change attitudes as compared to other methods. These findings are at the root of the movement to reduce the number of hours of lecture in the medical curriculum and replace them with the more "active" learning methods that are described in later chapters.

Despite these arguments, it has been reasoned that the lecture remains an effective and valuable format in medical education (Matheson, 2008). There are several compelling reasons why lectures have not disappeared from the curricula of most medical schools. First, lectures offer a great economy of faculty time since other formats (e.g., small group teaching) require a larger number of faculty per activity. Second, since this format can be as good as any other for the simple transfer of information, it still makes sense to lecture. Third, many faculty automatically think of lectures as the primary engine of the medical curriculum and really don't have much training, experience or desire to teach in other ways. Finally, students also take this view of the curriculum and often expect to receive lectures as the primary vehicle for knowledge transfer from the faculty.

The goal of this chapter is to present ways of organizing and presenting a large group presentation that goes beyond the traditional boundaries of the lecture format.

W.B. Jeffries (✉)
University of Vermont College of Medicine, Burlington, VT, USA

W.B. Jeffries, K.N. Huggett (eds.), *An Introduction to Medical Teaching*,
DOI 10.1007/978-90-481-3641-4_2, © Springer Science+Business Media B.V. 2010

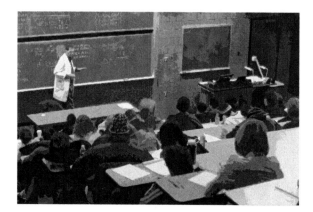

Our interest is in increasing student learning; this can be accomplished by modifying the format to introduce active learning methods. This will result in better learning, more engaged students and hopefully, better evaluations of your teaching. In this chapter, I will assume you have been given the assignment of presenting a lecture for the first time in a large course. The examples will be specific to medical school, but the lessons will apply to any teaching you will be called upon to make in a large group setting.

Creating an Environment that Supports Learning

Before considering the construction of the optimal large group presentation, it is useful to think about how students learn in this environment. Fuhrmann and Grasha (1983) describe well established ideas of cognitive function that explain how students learn in the lecture hall. First, students must be attentive and determine what to pay attention to. Thus it is your job to make the lecture interesting and facilitate student focus. This includes attention to presentation style, varying the format and eliminating distracters. Next, students must organize this information into a pattern that is understandable to them. The lecturer must therefore pay particular attention to organization, context and prior knowledge of the students. In other words, the presentation must be designed to lead the students to the achievement of the objectives. Finally, students must take the information that is stored in their short-term memory and add it to their existing long-term knowledge base through a process known as **rehearsal**. This implies that the lecturer should enable rehearsal to occur by reinforcing important points, summing up and introducing learning exercises that ensure that new information is applied in context. It also means that you must avoid introducing elements that confound the learning process (e.g., changing topics too quickly, introducing too much or irrelevant information, etc.).

Developing a Large Group Presentation

Context

Before planning your large group presentation it is a good idea to consider the role of each presentation in the course. Since many medical school courses are team-taught, your presentation is likely to be interrelated to those of one or more instructors. Thus preparation should begin with a thoughtful discussion between the lecturer and course director. First, you should discuss the overall course objectives and assessment methods. Within that framework, what is your presentation supposed to accomplish? Second, you should determine the depth and scope of your area of responsibility. What do you expect the students to have learned when the presentation is over? The answer to this question is best framed by writing out the objectives for the presentation (see below). Third, you should determine the relationship of the content assigned to you compared to that of the rest of the course. Is this topic related to other material in the course or curriculum? You should review the teaching materials presented by others on this topic to avoid gaps and redundancies of coverage. For example, if assigned a lecture on diabetes mellitus, you should consider how much carbohydrate metabolism should be included in your presentation. Fourth, you should become familiar with the instructional format of the course to ensure that your methods complement those used by others in the course. Within these boundaries, you should strive to include active learning methods to enhance student learning and maximize retention. In this vein, an appropriate question to ask is whether a lecture is the most appropriate format to use to cover the objectives. Other learning methods, found in later chapters in this book, may well prove to be the most optimal way to accomplish the course objectives. Assuming that this is not the case, planning for the lecture should continue as described below.

Purpose of the Presentation

Perhaps the most important question you can ask yourself when preparing a lecture for the first time is "what do I want my students to learn from this presentation?" Is it knowledge about a metabolic pathway? Is it how to perform a skill? It is how to critically interpret medical data? Is it to influence student attitudes about health policy? The answers to these questions help frame the objectives that you will construct to prepare the framework of the presentation. Further, they will influence how you present the material in the classroom. Table 2.1 shows some of the types of large group presentations that are classically used by medical teachers.

Development of the Content

If you are lecturing as part of a larger course, your broad goals and objectives are probably already defined. The content for your individual session is likely left up to

Table 2.1 Potential types of large group presentations and their purpose (Adapted from Newble and Cannon, 2001)

- *Presentation of information about a subject.* For example, a discussion of the etiology of heart failure.
- *Development of critical thinking skills.* For example, how to interpret epidemiological data about heart failure and apply that information to the diagnosis and treatment of a hypothetical patient.
- *Demonstration of a procedure or clinical approach.* For example, a demonstration of the use of the electrocardiogram in the diagnosis of heart ailments.
- *Construction an academic argument.* For example, influencing student attitudes regarding ethical policies of the distribution of donor hearts among transplant patients.

you. It is therefore initially useful to consider the subject broadly and reflect on the topic and its many aspects without regard to the limitations imposed by the course. Depending on your own preferences, the ideas can be in the form of lists of topics, concept maps, outcome lists, taxonomies, etc. An approach I find helpful is create a list of the possible areas of instruction needed to cover a particular broad topic, and then organize them into a logical order. For example, let's say you have been assigned to teach the pharmacology of drugs used to treat heart failure:

Heart Failure Drugs

1. Normal cardiac function.
2. Etiology of heart failure.

   a. Cellular.
   b. Organismal level.

3. Strategies to combat heart failure.
4. Drugs used to treat heart failure (repeat for each drug/class).

   a. Chemistry.
   b. Pharmacokinetics.
   c. Pharmacodynamics.

      i. Molecular and cellular effects.
      ii. Cardiac and hemodynamic effects.
      iii. Effects on other organs.

   d. Toxicity.
   e. Therapeutics.

When organized in this way, you will quickly discover several things about your presentation:

1. Your outline overlaps other areas of the course/curriculum. Students may have already been exposed to normal cardiac function and etiology of heart failure. As stated earlier, a discussion with the other faculty in the course will help set your boundaries. However, your outline is still helpful since it helps define the prerequisite knowledge that students must have to understand your lecture. The stage is set for seamlessly integrating your presentation into the rest of the course.
2. There is too much to cover! If you did it correctly, you have created an exhaustive outline of the topic. Aside from areas outside the topic areas as discussed in No. 1, your outline helps you understand/define the scope of knowledge you expect to cover in the lecture. If this topic is your particular area of expertise, you will be tempted to include a plethora of the latest research findings, new hypotheses about cardiac failure, drugs on the horizon, etc. However, if your learners are first year medical students, your focus should be on covering the basics, saving the advanced material for another audience. One of the most common mistakes I see among new faculty is an overestimation of what students need to know in lecture. An advantage of developing a topic list is to help identify the essentials.
3. There is more than one way to organize the material. The organization of topics need not be too refined at this stage. Thus you should just make sure at this point that all your ideas are captured. Later, you will organize the material based on your objectives and the styles of the course.
4. The process has uncovered gaps in your own knowledge about the subject. One of the benefits of teaching is that it helps you develop your own knowledge of various subjects. Your knowledge gaps will prompt you to read more on the topic or consult a colleague to bring yourself up to date. You should also familiarize yourself with the relevant chapters from the assigned textbooks for the course. This will help you decide what information needs to be emphasized in class vs. that which is best left to the student to learn from the textbook.

At this stage you can then go back and compare your ideas with the specific objectives assigned for your course and lecture. Are the objectives appropriate? Are they achievable in the time allotted? Are they in the need of modification? You will likely conclude that the objectives need to be modified in some way. For example, if the objectives are not achievable in the time allotted, you will have to prioritize information to be presented (i.e., that which will be deferred for student reading or other out-of-class exercise, etc.).

Development of the Lecture Plan

A well organized presentation improves learning and retention. What is the best way to organize a lecture? There is no best answer to this question; however, the organization should be dictated by several factors: the type of lecture (Table 2.1), the most logical sequence of information and the fostering of student attention, motivation and cognitive processing. Some common organizing principles are shown in Table 2.2.

Table 2.2 Ways to organize a large group presentation (adapted from McKeachie and Svinicki, 2006, p. 63)

- Inductive approaches
  - ○ Problem to solution (inductive approach)
  - ○ Clinical case to diagnosis and treatment
  - ○ Phenomenon to theory
- Deductive approaches
  - ○ Concept to application
  - ○ General discussion to specific cases
  - ○ Chaining of ideas (if A and B are true, then C must also be true)
- Time sequence (e.g., chronological stories)
- Pro vs. Con to solution
- Familiar to unfamiliar (what students know to what they don't know)

Inductive approaches imply that a real world example is first presented and then the case specifics are used to generalize and develop the underlying theories. For example, a case could be presented in which a patient has developed some of the signs and symptoms of heart failure. This would allow a discussion of the mechanisms by which the patient developed this condition, and the principles of treatment. This would lead to a discussion of the specific drugs. **Deductive approaches** begin with a discussion of the underlying concepts (e.g., cellular physiology of the heart, hemodynamics, etc.) which lead to the discussion of specific cases. Time sequencing can be an effective approach (e.g., the development of heart failure treatment as a series of scientific breakthroughs) since the telling of stories promotes retention. Similarly, presenting a **pro vs. con** framework promotes retention because the academic argument presented promotes engagement and retention. A **familiar to unfamiliar** progression helps establish for the students the context in which the material fits.

Obviously, several of these principles may be used within the same lecture and all of them can convey information and enhance student learning. The plan will also be dictated by the type of large group session that is needed. If the purpose of the session is primarily the delivery of information or demonstration of a procedure, the objectives should be ordered in a simple outline format. If the purpose is the development of critical thinking skills or construction of an argument, then the organization and sequence has to be less defined to allow adjustments during the teaching process. In this latter case the number of objectives also must be scaled back since the development of skills and attitudes needs time for development during the class period. Most importantly, regardless of the plan used, the students must be made aware of the organizational structure of the lecture to avoid confusion and enhance their ability to process information.

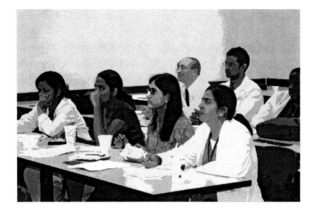

Presenting a Large Group Session

Using one or more of the formats outlined in the previous section, you should present a session that is designed to promote a learning-enabled environment. This means you will enhance attention, and use strategies to enhance cognitive function.

Planning the Beginning and the End

A great way to increase attention and instill student confidence is to have a well planned beginning to your lecture. In your first lecture, it is a good idea to introduce yourself and briefly discuss your larger role in the school (e.g., "I am a neuroscientist who researches the coordination of skeletal muscle movement by the brain, which is why I was chosen to discuss Parkinson's disease"). A brief, general outline of what will be covered is often the next step. It will aid learning if the students understand the framework of your talk in advance. It is convenient to use the learning objectives in the outline to clarify their importance. Depending on the type of lecture, the next step may be to address the gap between the student's current knowledge and that needed to understand the subject (e.g., "You all have an excellent understanding of carbohydrate metabolism. Today we will attempt to apply that knowledge to the understanding of the etiology of Diabetes Mellitus"). Alternatively, you may use this opportunity to introduce a case or open-ended problem, which will then form the basis for the content to come. The ending of the lecture should also be well planned. Here is it often best to summarize the most salient points of the lecture. This will aid in student rehearsal and provide them with a focus for later review. Time for final questions should also be allotted. This should include time for students to approach you immediately after the lecture in case they are uncomfortable asking their question in front of the class.

Projecting Enthusiasm

Students respond to the enthusiasm of the instructor with increased attentiveness (Bligh, 2000). There are many ways to project enthusiasm. The easiest is to move around the room and engage the audience. Conversely, the quickest way to classroom boredom is to use a monotone presentation and stand directly behind the podium. This is particularly true in a large lecture hall where students may not easily see your facial expressions. In this case it is important to get out from behind the podium and mingle with the audience. Make eye contact with specific students and vary your vocal expression. A trick that I use is to arrive early and scan the class photo (usually available from the course director or Office of Medical Education) to identify several students in the audience. During the lecture, you can call them by name and engage them specifically. Be careful to do this in a non-threatening manner! The judicious use of humor can also help maintain attention. If you are not comfortable with verbal witticisms, you can show a humorous cartoon. Relevant anecdotes also can enhance arousal and improve retention. Such overtures let the students see you are engaged and interested in a rapport with them. Student attention and engagement are bound to dramatically rise.

A note of caution is needed when discussing enthusiasm. Although enthusiasm does promote learning in the classroom, studies have shown that excellent engagement alone can be perceived as excellent learning by the students, irrespective of the actual value of the content (Ware and Williams, 1975). In these studies, a fictional "Dr. Fox" gave lectures with either a high degree of enthusiasm (movement, vocal emphasis, humor, etc.) or low enthusiasm (unexpressive, monotone delivery) and varying degrees of meaningful content. As expected, it was found that student learning was greatest in high enthusiasm/high content lectures. However, student ratings revealed that they considered a high enthusiasm teacher to be effective regardless of the level of content. Ware and Williams (1975) called this the "Dr. Fox Effect." Thus, students appreciate the entertainment value of the lecture and the instructor may come to an erroneous conclusion as to his/her effectiveness based on student feedback. One should always keep in mind that while enthusiasm is an effective tool to promote attention, challenging and meaningful content must also be introduced to produce student learning (Table 2.3).

Table 2.3 Tips for engagement

- Arrive early; stay late
- Move around the room, deliver various points from different locations
- Make eye contact with students
- Call students by name
- Make expressive gestures and body movements
- Vary the tone of your voice
- Ask questions
- Use humor
- Vary presentation style

Pacing and Density of Content

The speed at which material is introduced is a critical factor that influences learning. Often students are unfamiliar with material being introduced and must build their knowledge base over the course of the lecture. Studies of lecture pacing revealed that students hardly ever complain if the lecturer has a delivery that is too slow (Bligh, 2000, p. 223). On the other hand, if a lecture is paced too quickly, the ability of students to build concepts is overwhelmed and learning is impaired dramatically. The pace of delivery is directly related to the amount of information to be covered. In medical education it is common to see an instructor attempt to cover 80 or 90 detailed slides in a 50 min presentation. In this case, you can expect very little long term learning to occur. The speed necessary to deliver material of this density will reduce attention, depress cognition, inhibit effective note taking and decrease learning. Thus you must limit the amount of material in your presentation and focus it on major points to be remembered. If you have been assigned too much material and too little time it will be necessary to employ additional learning methods, such as assigned reading or homework problems to accomplish the learning objectives. The important thing to remember (and stress with the course director) is that simply speeding up the presentation is not a viable option.

Attention Span vs. Lecture Length

Some authors suggest that despite an enthusiastic presentation, student attention in the lecture hall can wane dramatically after only 10–15 min (summarized in Bligh, 2000 and McKeachie and Svinicki, 2006). While other authors suggest that this decline in attention span varies widely (Wilson and Korn, 2007), even highly motivated learners can begin to squirm in their seats and become distracted well before the lecture is over. Lecture length has another negative impact on learning: **interference**. Since there is a finite capacity to short-term memory, new material just learned can displace material learned just minutes earlier. This combination of reduced attention and interference can potentially create a gap in learning, particularly in the middle of the lecture. Fortunately there are measures you can take to prevent this. It has been shown that varying the format can restore attention. Further, providing opportunities for rehearsal of short-term memories into long-term learning can effectively combat interference. Therefore no more than 10–15 min should pass before summing up (which aids rehearsal) and introducing an active learning exercise to promote "hard coding" of student learning experiences. Some suggested exercises are included in the next section.

Getting Feedback

Even the best lecturers can lose their audience. I have witnessed well thought-out, enthusiastic lectures that were unfortunately delivered at a level well beyond the student's learning capacity. Thus it is imperative to obtain feedback from your learners during the presentation to determine that they are actually following and comprehending your presentation. The easiest way to get this information is to ask at the end of each major point if there are any questions.

This often elicits no response, especially in the large lecture hall. This may be because everyone understands, or some students may be too intimidated in the presence of their peers to admit that they don't understand something. One of the ways to approach this challenge is to create buzz groups (see next section) which can be used to identify the "muddiest point." Another newer solution is via the use of an audience response system. This system, described in Chapter 9, can elicit anonymous answers to questions posed by you during lecture. This approach serves a dual purpose. First, you can obtain real-time feedback as to whether students comprehend your lecture. Second, you are allowing rehearsal of the most important concepts during lecture, which should dramatically enhance retention.

Handouts

Studies have shown that note-taking increases learning and retention of the material presented in large group formats. Thus it is a good idea to prepare handouts that lend themselves to note taking and reinforcement of the lessons given in class. A familiar format is a general outline that can be filled in with specifics during the lecture. Another common format is to provide an exact copy of your presentation slides in paper or electronic form to the students. This allows students to annotate your presentation in the lecture hall. Both of these formats are easily posted into online content management systems and allow students to use their computers to take detailed, typed notes on your presentation. One should beware three things when preparing handouts for use in class. First, make sure that you have not provided too much information, such as long, detailed bullet points. This discourages note taking and encourages the instructor to read them off in the lecture, reducing engagement. Second, make sure that slides that are easily seen when projected are also easily read when printed. Slides featuring detailed histology can become amorphous smudges, graph legends can disappear and complex biochemical reactions can be undecipherable when rendered as six black and white images per page. Thus, it is worth taking the time to look over how the handout of your presentation will look before entering the lecture hall. Finally, ensure that you have secured copyright permissions for figures and materials you will include in your handouts. Once in the student's hands, these documents fall into the public domain and you are responsible for the content in them.

Audiovisual Materials

Audiovisual materials introduced in a large group presentation should complement the presentation and promote active learning. The most common presentation method in large group settings is the "slide show," in which the instructor can project text and images to illustrate the important points of the lecture. The physical slide has given way to electronic presentation formats, most commonly Microsoft PowerPoint. Some tips for an effective slide show can be found in Table 2.4. More specific guidelines for use of PowerPoint can be found in Chapter 9.

Table 2.4 Effective slide presentations

- Avoid dark background with white letters. This requires lower room lighting, which encourages dozing.
- Don't put too much information on a single slide. The number of bullet points should not exceed 4–5. The font size should be as large as possible, at least 18 pt.
- Ensure that figures are legible when projected.
- Do not put conflicting information formats on a single slide (e.g., a graph with bullet point explanation).
- Bullet points should not be detailed sentences. Rather, they should be heading names that allow for expansion in class.
- Allow 2–3 min per slide.
- Allow for other educational elements to be included in the presentation. A single lecture of 50 PowerPoint slides is a sure way to lose the student's attention.

Other audiovisual materials can include videos, demonstrations, white or black board, models, etc. The key to the use of these materials is that they are relevant, visible at a distance, and easily comprehended in the lecture hall. With regard to this latter point, I recall a colleague who developed a detailed animation of a physiological process for presentation in class, but the students who viewed it could not comprehend its complexity in the allotted time. Audiovisual materials should help explain things, not provide barriers to understanding.

Active Learning Methods in the Lecture Hall

As stated previously, a key to increasing learning in the large group setting is involving the students with active rather than passive methods. When introducing active learning methods into the lecture hall, you may meet some resistance. Some students do not understand the need for active learning methods. A question you may sometimes get is "why can't you just tell us what we need to remember for the exam?" In this case you should state that the purpose of the presentation is to learn about the material IN THE CLASSROOM. Tell them that valid educational data show that sitting for an hour just listening is not the best way to learn. Thus other elements of active learning MUST be incorporated into the hour. Finally, you must ensure that your assessment questions on examinations require more than just rote memorization. If students are made aware of this, there will be great interest in active learning in the classroom. Students who initially disapproved of these techniques have regaled me years later with stories about how they still remember lecture points solidified by active learning methods. In this section I will introduce some ideas for

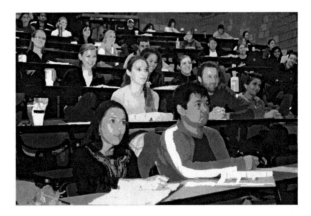

incorporating active learning into a large group session. The list is not exhaustive, but is intended to start you in a search for the best methods to complement your own presentation style.

Lecture Respites

The simplest way to promote student learning during a lecture is to provide a short respite from lecture. This can be done every 10–15 min to maintain student arousal. One way is to say "at this point I will stop for a **note check**. I want you to review your notes and then ask me questions if needed." This simple device allows students to begin to make sense of the lecture, clarify points they don't understand, and process the information into long-term memory. You can help the process along by suggesting areas to focus on in their brief review, or present or ask a question yourself for them to go and answer from their notes. The solitary review should last only about a minute, to discourage social chatting with neighbors.

Small Group Activities

The best way to overcome the limitations of a large group is to break up the class into smaller units that can engage in other activities. **Buzz groups** are a form of peer learning that can be introduced into any large group presentation. The instructor poses a problem, and then divides the class in groups of about four students each to quickly solve it. In my lectures I simply ask the students to turn to their neighbors and discuss the problem. After a short interval (2–3 min) the instructor calls on a reporter from each group to present their answer. The question can be subdivided so that different groups have different parts of the question, which can promote a class-wide discussion to synthesize the best solution. Further questions can be introduced during the discussion by the instructor to promote further discussion. I sometimes create impromptu buzz groups if I feel that the class is having difficulty understanding a concept. The buzz group format is quite adaptable and can occupy just a few minutes or an extended time as needed. A variant of the buzz group is the "**Think-Pair-Share**" or "**Pair discussion**." Here students work on a problem or discussion question of limited complexity by themselves for 1–5 min (**think**), then form a working pair with their nearest neighbor (**pair**). The discussion time allotted is also short (about 3–5 min), and the instructor calls on a limited number of pairs to report and discuss their answer (**share**). Despite the limited discussion period, all students work on the problem with a peer and derive benefits from actively applying their new knowledge in this format. The pair discussion format can also be combined with the note check strategy described above in which students determine if they have missed anything, discuss the salient points and ensure that they both agree on what was important.

Reading or problem solving activities can also be attempted in a large group setting. There are many variations to this format, but it is usually the assignment of a specific reading, viewing a video vignette or problem-solving task. Students complete the tasks individually for a defined period of time, then break into pairs or small groups for discussion and resolution of problems. Then the groups report to the large group during a general large group discussion facilitated by the instructor. There are many possible variants to this scenario.

Classroom Survey Techniques

Classroom survey techniques are methods to poll the class about their preferences on certain topics or answers to questions during the session. This can be done by eliciting a simple show of hands, by holding up numbered cards or by use of sophisticated audience response systems as described in Chapter 9. This format can create a lively and interactive environment to promote learning in a large group. The most common approach to the method is to periodically ask the students a multiple choice question and to quickly tally the answers from the class. There are tangible benefits to both the instructor and the student. The instructor receives instant feedback as to the comprehension of the class and can adjust the content and pace of the lecture accordingly. Disparate answers can also be used to generate a class discussion. For the student, attentiveness is improved and knowledge gained during the lecture is directly applied to promote long-term retention. Use of an automated audience response system can greatly facilitate this process. In addition to instant feedback, the audience response system offers the advantage of anonymous responses, integration with presentation software, individual tracking and grading of responses and immediate graphical display of the results. When using any classroom survey technique, the instructor must be prepared to alter the course of the presentation based on the level of comprehension of the students. A final use of classroom survey techniques worth discussing is for assessment. Short quizzes can be introduced at the end of lectures to reinforce learning. Conversely, quizzes can be introduced at the beginning of each lecture to assess prior knowledge or to ensure completion of the reading assignment.

Two-Minute Paper

The two-minute paper or "half sheet response" is an effective way for students to synthesize the knowledge gained during the large group session (McKeachie and Svinicki, 2006, p. 256). Typically, the students are asked to take 2 min at the end of class to produce a short essay explaining the most salient point(s) of the lecture. Other topics that could be tasked include "Give an example of this concept" or "discuss treatment options for this disease," etc. This aids in retention and understanding of the material. The essay can be for self evaluation or the instructor can collect them for grading. A variant is where the instructor stops the class and asks them to produce a two-minute essay on an assigned topic that relates to the lecture material.

Games

Some faculty are able to introduce active learning in students by catering to their competitive nature. In the game format, quiz questions are introduced and student teams compete to answer them. Scores may be kept and nominal prizes may even be awarded to the best teams. There are many variations to this format. Small competitions can be held during the last 5 min of the session, or entire sessions can be given over to review a course section via this approach. The biggest advantage of the game approach is that it creates a fun, energy filled environment for learning. The primary disadvantages are the time it takes to conduct the sessions and the loss of focus that can occur in the game environment.

Team-Based Learning

Team-Based Learning (TBL) is a large group peer teaching format that focuses on the application of student knowledge to problems. Students in the large group setting are divided into teams of 5–8 students, arranged at tables in a large room. In this format students are assigned a reading or other activity, then meet as a group to various questions posed by the faculty facilitator. The advantage of TBL is it uses the strength of peer teaching in a well controlled format that ensures coverage of the learning objectives. The disadvantage of this approach is that it requires specific classroom configurations and a course or curriculum-wide commitment to successfully implement it. A full discussion of TBL can be found in Chapter 5.

A Final Word

Developing and delivering an effective lecture can be a daunting challenge. It is important to review the feedback gained from students and peers and to continue to improve the quality and the amount of learning that takes place in your sessions.

Table 2.5 Common mistakes to avoid in large group teaching

- Lack of engagement: monotone presentation from behind the podium
- Information overload: too many slides, too fast paced, too many objectives
- Poorly thought out beginning and ending
- Simply reading bullet points off of the slides
- Inadequate knowledge of context of your presentation: Gaps, redundancies and conflicting information
- No time for assimilation and reflection
- Not knowing your learners: Teaching is too elementary or beyond their comprehension
- Entertaining, but not informative: Beware the Dr. Fox effect!

Table 2.5 summarizes some of the common pitfalls that can befall even the most experienced lecturers. Further information on diagnosing lecture problems can be found in a humorous but informative paper by McLaughlin and Mandin (2001). Chapter 12 discusses in detail how to use evaluation data to improve your teaching.

Hopefully this chapter has provided both a framework for engaging students actively in the large group setting and a way of avoiding common mistakes. Additional resources are provided below to provide an in-depth treatment of this topic.

References

Bligh DA (2000) What's the use of lectures? Jossey-Bass, New York.

Matheson C (2008) The educational value and effectiveness of lectures. The Clinical Teacher 5: 219–221.

McKeachie WJ, Svinicki M (2006) McKeachie's teaching tips. Strategies, research, and theory for college and university teachers. Houghton Mifflin, Boston, MA.

McLaughlin K, Mandin H (2001) A schematic approach to diagnosing and resolving lecturalgia. Medical Education 35: 1135–1142.

Newble D, Cannon R (2001) A handbook for medical teachers, 4th ed. Kluwer Academic Publishers, Dodrecht, The Netherlands.

Fuhrmann B, Grasha A (1983) A Practical handbook for college teachers. Little, Brown and Company, Boston.

Ware JE, Williams RG (1975) The Dr. Fox effect: A study of lecturer effectiveness and ratings of instruction. Journal of Medical Education 50: 149–156.

Wilson K, Korn JH (2007) Attention during lectures: Beyond ten minutes. Teaching of Psychology 34(2): 85–89.

Chapter 3
Teaching in Small Groups

Kathryn N. Huggett

There are many unique benefits to teaching and learning in small groups. Recognizing this, many medical schools have increased the amount of time devoted to small group learning. Very few faculty members, however, have received instruction for leading small groups. This has contributed to misperceptions about the value of small group learning. It also explains why many faculty members do not feel confident teaching in this setting. Teaching in small groups can be satisfying and even inspiring, but it can also be time consuming and dispiriting when difficulties arise. To ensure effective small group teaching, you must first understand the purpose for the small group and then select activities for the group that will enable learners to achieve the learning objectives. Understanding both your role as the teacher and the dynamics of the group will help you foster participation among group members.

Reasons for Teaching in Small Groups

There are many advantages to teaching in small groups. The smaller number of participants means that you will have an opportunity to know your students' names and become familiar with their knowledge, learning styles, and prior learning experiences. As the course progresses, you will be able to conduct ongoing assessment, both formal and informal, of learners' comprehension and application of the course content. This will enhance your efforts to target your teaching strategies. Learners in a small group benefit because they have increased contact time with their instructor. You will find learners are more comfortable asking questions during small group sessions than larger lectures.

There are significant educational outcomes associated with teaching and learning in small groups. The small number of learners promotes engagement between learners, the instructor, and the content. You will be able to introduce activities that require learners to move beyond the recall and recognition of concepts. When teaching in small groups, you can ask learners to employ higher-order thinking skills

K.N. Huggett (✉)
Creighton University School of Medicine, Omaha, NE, USA

W.B. Jeffries, K.N. Huggett (eds.), *An Introduction to Medical Teaching*,
DOI 10.1007/978-90-481-3641-4_3, © Springer Science+Business Media B.V. 2010

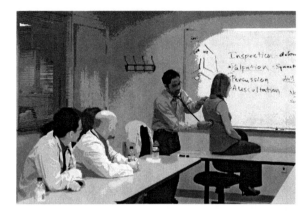

such as analysis, reasoning, and criticism. To do this, you might create opportunities for learners to demonstrate problem-solving skills. These activities will allow you to assess if your learners are able to apply new knowledge and concepts. Similarly, the small group provides a venue for learners to rehearse material they have read or learned in lectures. They can pose questions about the material, discuss inconsistencies, and propose applications of the material. This will help learners to see and understand the connections between the material in your course and others in their area of study. As the small group facilitator, you can provide learners with information about the context for the material and its relevance. This will also assist learners in understanding and applying new knowledge.

Small groups offer two additional educational outcomes. First, the small size and increased engagement of the group promote reflection on learning. Recognizing what you have learned, what you do not know, and what you still need to know is essential to becoming a professional. This is the foundation of lifelong learning, and you can model this for your learners. In addition to fostering reflection on learning, small groups provide learners with opportunities to develop the interpersonal skills necessary to work in a group or team setting. This is becoming more important as health care is increasingly provided by teams of diverse professionals. Participation in small groups can improve skills in active listening, presentation, negotiation, group leadership, and cooperative problem solving.

Definition of Small Group Teaching

Teaching and learning can occur anywhere, but some learning objectives are best achieved by small group teaching. Small groups are often used to complement lecture-based courses. When this occurs, the small group meets to discuss the lectures or readings. Small groups are also ideal for working through cases that integrate material from the lectures or other required courses. Small group teaching and learning also occur in problem-based curricula and laboratory courses. Each of these small group activities presents unique considerations for planning and teaching, and will be discussed elsewhere in this book.

The size of small groups can vary considerably in medical education. Research has demonstrated that groups composed of five to eight learners are the optimal size. However, limitations posed by physical space and faculty availability lead many medical schools to organize small groups with more than eight learners.

The size of the group is not the only determinant of small group teaching. In medical education it is not unusual to find learners in a small group session listening to a lecture given by the instructor. This is not small group teaching. Newble and Cannon (2001) cite three important characteristics of small group teaching:

- Active participation.
- Purposeful activity.
- Face-to-face contact.

Active Participation

To realize the educational benefits of small group teaching, it is essential that all members of the group participate. The small group size will ensure there is time and opportunity for all learners to contribute to the discussion or activity. This is important because you will want to assess each learner's development in knowledge and understanding. Greater participation among all group members also ensures sufficient opportunities for learners to hone their communication and team skills. If the group is larger than eight learners, you can still use small group teaching methods, but will need to be both creative and deliberate in planning the activities. Some of the techniques for teaching in small groups can be accomplished successfully if you create multiple subgroups within the existing small group.

Purposeful Activity

We have all had the unpleasant experience of participating in a meeting or small group session where there is no agenda or plan for the activity. The lack of purpose creates frustration and anxiety, and contributes to the feeling that our time was misspent. This is not unlike the experience learners have when small group teaching is not organized around purposeful activity. The purpose, or goal, you create for each session may be broad, but then the session and discussion should be organized to accomplish this goal. In addition to determining the content focus of the session, you will also want to think about the other learning outcomes that can be achieved during the session, such as critical appraisal of the literature or team negotiation. Too much activity can also become a problem, especially if it limits participation by all group members. Developing a plan for each session will help ensure that learners remain engaged and that the goals of the session are met. A small group session plan is also helpful for small group leaders who are less experienced or less skilled in small group teaching. The plan will provide guidance on how to structure the session activities and manage time effectively.

Face-to-Face Contact

While recent advances in instructional technology have fostered effective strategies for online or e-learning, the type of small group teaching described in this chapter requires face-to-face contact. A synchronous, or "real-time," discussion requires that learners demonstrate presentation skills or work collaboratively to apply knowledge and solve a new problem. As the instructor, you will be able to observe these skills and also learners' non-verbal communication skills such as eye contact and posture. Likewise, learners need to be able to see the other members of their group, and it may be necessary to reconfigure the room so this can occur. If possible, reserve seminar-style rooms or rooms with furniture that can be re-arranged easily.

Preparing for the Small Group Session

Preparing for small group teaching begins like preparing for any other type of teaching. First, determine the learning objectives for the session. One way to do this is to write a list of outcomes, where each statement begins "By the end of this session, learners will be able to. . ." As you fill in the blank with a knowledge, skill or attitude objective, remember that the small group session is an appropriate place to ask learners to demonstrate higher-order thinking skills such as reasoning and critical appraisal. Taxonomies, such as those developed by Bloom (1956) and revised by Anderson et al. (2001), provide guidance on classifying learning objectives. Consult Chapter 1 of this book for a review of learning objectives and taxonomies of thinking skills, including an overview of a taxonomy developed by Quellmaz (Stiggins et al., 1988). Review your list of objectives periodically, and ask yourself if the small group is the best place to teach and learn each objective.

After you have determined the learning objectives for the session, review the characteristics of the learners enrolled in the small group. Is this course their first introduction to the subject matter? Can you assume they have all completed similar core courses or prerequisites? The answers to these questions will help you determine expectations for their participation. Are you acquainted with the learners already? Are they acquainted with each other? This is important to know before asking learners to work collaboratively or discuss sensitive topics.

The next step in planning the small group session is to determine the structure for the session. First, review the amount of time allotted for the session and the total number of sessions for the topic and course. Then establish which objectives will be addressed in each session. If you are responsible for planning a session within a series of small group sessions, review your colleagues' plans to ensure your coverage of the content is complementary and not redundant. Next, determine the appropriate activity for teaching and learning the objectives. For example, you might begin the session by inviting learners to discuss points that were unclear in the recent lecture. Then the session might continue with discussion of a case and conclude with time for learners to reflect on the case and ask questions. To ensure that you accomplish all planned activities within the allotted amount of time, develop an agenda for each session. An example of an agenda for a small group discussion session in a medical ethics course is illustrated in Table 3.1.

Table 3.1 Agenda for a small group session in a medical ethics course

Activity	Time (min)
Attendance and announcements	5
Student presentation of ethics case	10
Presenters identify 2 unresolved ethical questions	5
Group discussion of the case and questions	20
Student presentation of case and commentaries from textbook	10
Group discussion of the case and commentaries	20
Wrap-up and review of deadlines for upcoming assignments	5
Total session time	75

Do not feel that the agenda or schedule cannot be changed, however. You will need to adapt the plan as the session unfolds. Some tasks may require less time than you estimated and it will be appropriate to begin the next activity earlier than planned. During some sessions, you may need to re-allocate time to clarify difficult concepts or address questions that arise. The outline should be a guide and not a rigid schedule. Over time, you will feel more comfortable adapting the schedule.

Leading the Small Group Session

Thoughtful preparation before teaching small groups will lead to well-organized sessions that are integrated into the curriculum for the course. However, careful planning can only ensure part of the success of teaching in small groups. As a small group facilitator, you will soon find that your leadership and the dynamics of the group are critical elements.

Attributes of an Effective Small group Teacher

Effective small group teachers are well prepared for each session and are acquainted with goals and objectives for the entire course. Take time to become familiar with the lecture topics in the course, especially those that relate to the cases or topics discussed in the small group session. The time you spend preparing in advance of each small group will improve the organization and flow of each session. You may also find you spend less time on learners' questions about the administrative details

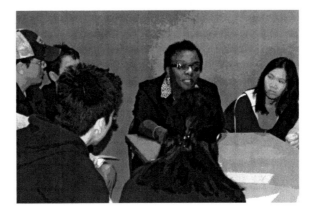

of the course and more time on learning. How you conduct yourself during the session may be even more important than how much you prepare. Your primary focus is the learner, and not the content or activity. Effective small group teachers demonstrate interest in and respect for their learners. One way to do this is to introduce yourself at the first session, and briefly tell learners about your role in the course or other responsibilities in medical education. Also, remember to let learners know how to reach you if they have questions outside of the small group session. Another way to demonstrate respect for your learners is to recognize that each small group will be composed of learners with different personality types and learning styles. These shape learners' responses to the tasks and roles that are assigned within the group. Two sources for information about personality types are the Myers-Briggs Type Indicator (1995) and Keirsey Temperament Sorter (1998). Both instruments provide insight into an individual's predispositions and attitudes. These tests do not assess ability or psychological traits; instead, results from these profiles can help to explain how individuals differ when making decisions or obtaining new information. To better understand differences in individuals' preferences for learning, consult David Kolb's Learning Styles Inventory (LSI) (1984). The LSI is a well-known model of learning styles based upon a cycle of learning that describes how all people learn. Kolb's theory of experiential learning will be described in greater detail in Chapter 7.

While effective small group teachers appreciate the differences among learners, they also understand that their own personality type and learning preferences may differ from those of their students. Our preferences even influence our leadership style in the small group setting. For example, some teachers are highly-skilled at lecturing to large groups. They may prefer to teach and learn in this type of environment where attention is focused on the individual instructor and there is minimal interaction with the group. For this individual, moving to the interactive, small-group setting can be challenging. It is not unusual for this type of teacher to revert to lecturing within the small group, especially if they perceive group activity as difficult to manage. Acknowledging these preferences for teaching and learning will help you to recognize when your own style begins to overshadow the learner-centered approach.

Effective small group teachers also promote a learner-centered approach to small group teaching by providing frequent, formative feedback. This type of feedback helps learners to assess their progress and make changes while the course is still in progress. Feedback should be specific so that learners recognize which element of their performance should be improved or, in the case of positive feedback, continued. Specific examples and constructive suggestions for improvement will enhance the quality of feedback.

Conditions for an Effective Small Group Session

Successful small group sessions rarely occur simply because of an enthusiastic teacher or motivated learners. Effective, learner-centered groups require multiple conditions for success. First, each group should agree upon ground rules such as no late arrivals or criticism during idea-generating activities. If students are new to small group learning, you may want to explain that all learners have a right to participate, but they can pass or occasionally request assistance from a classmate. Likewise, you may want to discuss rules to limit speaking too frequently during the sessions. These basic rules will help to promote respect among group members and develop group cohesion. If you engage learners in determining expectations for peer behavior, you will find they are more invested in the group and more likely to adhere to the group's norms for behavior. Second, each small group should discuss clear guidelines for participation and assessment. As the small group teacher, you should explain your expectations for participation and how this contributes to the evaluation of learners' performance. When learners are confused about the criteria for assessment, they may become anxious and less willing to participate. Take time to clarify the roles that learners will play in the small group, such as presenter or reporter, and explain how often learners will change roles. Likewise, explain to learners which resources they are responsible for bringing to the session so that they arrive prepared. Small group sessions are less likely to become unfocused or unproductive when learners are prepared and informed about the purpose and expectations for the session.

Finally, small groups generally flourish in an environment that is cooperative and collaborative, rather than competitive. While occasional friendly competition, such as a quiz-show activity, might engage the group and promote collegiality, a pervasive environment of cut-throat competition will stifle participation. As a small group teacher, you can develop activities that require collaboration and should intervene when an overly competitive learner seeks control of the session or resources.

Understanding Group Dynamics

Small groups in medical education share many characteristics with small groups or teams organized for other professional purposes. Scholtes et al. (2000), building upon earlier work by Bruce Tuckman (1965), describe a four-stage process that all groups undergo. This model is useful for anticipating learners' attitudes and behaviors in your small group. In the first stage, called **forming**, group members feel excitement, anticipation and optimism. Some learners may also experience anxiety or suspicion about the work ahead. Scholtes encourages leaders to help the group members become acquainted and develop rules during the forming stage. In the second stage, **storming**, learners may exhibit resistance to tasks or express concern about excessive work. Arguments between group members may arise. The effective small group teacher will help learners resolve these issues. In the third stage, **norming**, groups demonstrate acceptance of small group members. A developing sense of cohesion fosters discussion and constructive criticism. During this stage, effective small group teachers will promote collaboration. The final stage, **performing**, is characterized by the group's ability to work through problems. Sholtes notes that group members now have a better understanding of each others' strengths and weaknesses. The effective small group teacher will monitor progress and provide feedback during this stage. Groups will differ in how much time they spend in each stage of the process, but will ideally spend most of their time in the latter stages. As the small group teacher, you can observe the group and facilitate appropriate transitions between stages.

Small Group Discussion Methods

There are many approaches to teaching in small groups but the most successful ones are organized around a purposeful activity. In medical education, the structured case discussion is a common approach. Learners present a patient case and then work together to accomplish tasks such as developing a diagnosis and management plan. As described earlier in Table 3.1, a structured case discussion session typically allows the majority of time for individual learner presentations and group discussion. A limited amount of time is allocated for the small group leader to open and conclude the session and, as needed, clarify aspects of the case that are unclear. The structured approach to the case discussion means that time is allocated for each task. This ensures that the discussion is organized and stays on course.

While the case is a common stimulus for small group discussion in the health sciences, there are other materials that can be used to organize or initiate discussion. Examples of stimulus material include:

- A brief audio or video presentation.
- Visual material pertinent to the discussion (e.g., diagnostic images or charts).
- Material available via the Internet.
- A journal article or other thought-provoking written material.
- A real or standardized patient.

- Observation of a role play.
- A "one minute paper" that learners write and then share.
- A brief multiple choice test.

Variations in Small Group Teaching

In addition to case discussion, there are other methods that can be used in teaching small groups. When you prepare to teach in a small group setting, consider the purpose or goal for the session, and then select a technique that is best suited to achieving the learning objectives. Sometimes it is useful to introduce a different technique to promote learner interest and engagement.

1. *One-to-one discussion*: The one-to-one discussion is easy to facilitate and effective for many topics. To use this technique, organize the group into pairs. As the small group teacher, you can participate in this activity as well. One member of each pair should talk on the assigned topic for 3–5 minutes, without interruption. The roles are then reversed and the other member of the pair becomes the discussant. You may need to remind the group periodically that questions and comments should be held until later in the session. After the pairs have concluded their one-to-one discussion, the group reconvenes and each person provides a brief summary of the comments made by their partner. This technique helps learners to develop listening, summarization, and presentation skills. The one-to-one discussion is effective as an introductory ice breaker, where learners use the discussion and presentation time to meet and learn more about their colleagues. This small group technique is also valuable for discussing topics that are emotionally-charged or controversial. By assigning learners to pairs and enforcing the time limit, everyone in the group will have an opportunity to participate. This approach will also ensure that garrulous or opinionated learners do not take control of the session.
2. *Buzz groups*: This small group discussion technique is used to engage learners and re-energize the group. To initiate the buzz group, pose a question and ask learners to discuss their responses in pairs or groups no larger than four learners. The room will soon be buzzing with conversation. This technique is useful for making a transition from one discussion task to another, or for encouraging learners to share ideas or concerns they might be reluctant to share with the entire group. As a small group teacher, your role is to facilitate the process and use the buzz group as a source of informal feedback about learners' understanding of the course material.
3. *Snowballing group discussion*: The snowballing group discussion is a variation on buzz groups and is named for the progression of activities during the session. With each step in the sequence, the size of group increases. Learners begin by working individually, then in pairs, and then in small groups. The session concludes with time for reporting back to the entire group. Snowballing group discussions are useful because they foster interaction among all members of the group. This discussion technique also provides time for all learners to complete

their individual preparation before working with other group members. The one drawback is that learners may tire of the topic or task, so you should plan to vary the task or increase complexity with each step.

4. *Group round*: The purpose of this small group discussion technique is to involve everyone in the group and generate interest in a topic. Each learner provides a brief response, no more than one minute, before moving on to the next learner. There are several ways to determine the order in which learners will participate. For consistency and efficiency, the teacher or group can determine the order at the beginning of the session. For a more spontaneous approach, the learner who is speaking can select the next learner, and this continues until all members of the group have participated. This method will generate more interest and engagement than the former two approaches. Learners may be permitted to pass at least one time during the group round.

5. *Brainstorming*: Brainstorming sessions are used to produce a large number of creative solutions or hypotheses in a short amount of time. This technique is also effective for encouraging learners to recall material learned at an earlier time. After a question or topic is identified, learners are asked to name ideas as they think of them. The group is forbidden to critique the ideas until after the brainstorming session has closed. Brainstorming promotes interaction within the group, but there are limitations to this strategy. For example, some learners may require more processing time to generate new ideas, and may not feel like they have much to contribute to the session until afterwards. Another potential problem is that some learners may choose not to participate. These "social loafers" may not have prepared sufficiently, and will gladly let others conduct the work of the group.

6. *Role-playing*: This strategy is particularly useful for learning and practicing communication skills such as interviewing or history taking. For some role-play sessions, it is possible to ask learners to play all of the roles (e.g., physician or patient) in the case or simulated encounter. For more advanced role-plays, including those that cover sensitive topics, it may be more appropriate to recruit and train standardized, actor patients. An example of an agenda for a role-playing session used in a course on interviewing skills is illustrated in Table 3.2.

Table 3.2 Agenda for a role-playing session with 2 practice interviews

	Activity
1	Attendance and announcements
2	Overview of the learning objectives and skills to be assessed during the interviewing session
3	Student 1 exits the room and waits for his/her interview
4	Student 2 interviews the Standardized Patient
5	The group provides feedback to Student 2
6	Student 1 interviews the Standardized Patient
7	The group provides feedback to Student 1
8	Wrap-up and review of key learning objectives

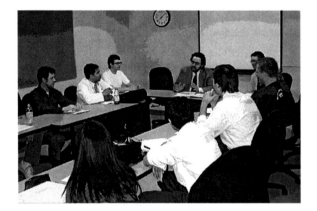

Small Group Teaching and Technology

Technologies such as SMART^{TM} boards, video, web-based reference materials, computer exercises, conferencing and simulation can enhance small group learning and promote purposeful activity. Educational technologies have also made it easier for learners and teachers to communicate and share information outside of scheduled small group sessions. These technologies will be discussed in greater detail in Chapter 9, but it is worth noting that online communities, such as blogs, wikis, and discussion boards, can be used to enhance the work of a face-to-face small group. For example, you might ask learners in your small group to maintain a blog and post brief reflections or questions after sessions that are particularly challenging. Unlike a traditional journal, the blog can include hyperlinks to other Web-based content, and can be accessed easily by others.

Evaluation of Small Group Participation and Learning

Evaluating small group participation and learning sends a message to learners that the activity is a meaningful part of the curriculum. Learners are also more likely to participate and prepare for the session if they know their contribution will count. Criteria for assessing participation should be explicit. When possible, invite small group learners to participate in determining some of these criteria so they feel responsible for their learning and the success of the group. This should occur soon after the course begins, often at the time the group establishes rules and norms. Examples of criteria to assess participation include these expectations of the student:

- Contributes to the discussion with evidence of preparation.
- Provides comparative assessments.
- Builds upon others' contributions.
- Willing to listen to others.
- Respects different viewpoints.

- Provides constructive criticism.
- Helps to summarize the discussion.

When establishing the criteria for small group participation, take care to not create a high-stakes environment. If learners are anxious about participation, they will not participate fully. You may also need to remind the group periodically about rules or norms to prevent the same learners from dominating the discussion.

Evaluation of Small Group Teaching

Teaching in small groups, like any teaching activity, will benefit from evaluation by learners and faculty. To evaluate your teaching, you will need to collect information that accurately describes the activity and then make a judgment about this information. Evaluation of teaching is discussed in greater detail in Chapter 12, but a few points specific to teaching in small groups merit attention here.

Informal Evaluation

Informal, ongoing evaluation can be useful for identifying aspects of the small group experience that detract from learning but can be corrected while the course is still in session. Examples of methods to collect informal evaluation data include brief online surveys; fast feedback cards collected at the end of a session; and periodic group debriefings.

Formal Evaluation

Formal evaluation of small group teaching should draw upon multiple sources of data and seek to promote validity and reliability. One source of data is student evaluations or questionnaires. Most departments or schools provide these, and items typically address topics such as the small group instructor's ability to facilitate the group, contribution of small group activities to improving understanding of the material, quality of resource materials, workload or amount of material covered, organization of the small group activities, and feedback on learning. Peer review of teaching is another source of valuable data. Colleagues who are knowledgeable about the subject can observe and evaluate how well the small group sessions promote discussion and understanding of key concepts. Colleagues who are not content experts can provide helpful insight into group dynamics and your skills as a facilitator. If your school does not provide resources for peer review of teaching, consult Chism's (2007) comprehensive guide to peer review of teaching. This includes resources and observation forms to ensure standardized assessment. A third source of data is video recordings of small group sessions. Some small group instructors find it helpful to review recordings, sometimes with the assistance of an educational consultant or trusted colleague, to identify aspects of teaching that are effective or require improvement. While all of these methods can provide useful data, be careful to ensure reliability by examining your teaching on multiple occasions. The interactive and personal nature of small group teaching makes it rewarding, but also highly variable.

References

Anderson LW, Krathwohl DR (eds), Airasian PW, Cruikshank KA, Mayer RE, Pintrich PR, Raths J, Wittrock MC (2001) A taxonomy for learning, teaching, and assessing: A revision of Bloom's Taxonomy of Educational Objectives (Complete edition). Longman, New York.
Bloom BS (ed), Engelhart MD, Furst EJ, Hill WH, Krathwohl DR (1956) Taxonomy of educational objectives: The classification of educational goals. Handbook 1: Cognitive domain. David McKay, New York.
Chism N (2007) Peer review of teaching. Anker Publishing Co, Bolton, MA.
Keirsey D (1998) Please understand me II: Temperament, character, intelligence. Prometheus Nemesis Book Company, Del Mar, CA.
Kolb DA (1984) Experiential learning: Experience as the source of learning and development. Prentice-Hall, Englewood Cliffs, NJ.
Myers IB, Myers PB (1995) Gifts differing: Understanding personality type. Davies-Black Publishing, Mountain View, CA.
Newble D, Cannon R (2001) A handbook for medical teachers, 4th ed. Kluwer Academic Publishers, Dodrecht, The Netherlands.
Scholtes PR, Joiner BL, Joiner BJ (2000) The TEAM handbook. Oriel, Inc, Madison, WI.
Stiggins RJ, Rubel E, Quellmalz E (1988) Measuring thinking skills in the classroom, rev ed. National Education Assn Professional Library, West Haven, CT.
Tuckman B (1965) Developmental sequence in small groups. Psychological Bulletin 63: 384–399.

For Further Reading

For a concise summary of recommendations for teaching in small groups, review

> Jacques D (2003) ABC of teaching and learning in medicine: Teaching small groups. British Medical Journal 326: 492–494.

For an in-depth examination of the concepts and techniques introduced in this chapter, consult

> Westberg J, Jason H (1996) Fostering learning in small groups: A practical guide. Springer, New York.

For further reading on the conditions for establishing effective small groups, read

> Wlodkowski RJ (1999) Enhancing adult motivation to learn. Jossey-Bass, San Francisco, CA.

Chapter 4
Problem-Based Learning

Mark A. Albanese

Problem-based learning (PBL) was created at McMaster University almost 40 years ago. It has changed medical education in ways that would not have been foreseen. It has supplanted the traditional lecture-based learning model in many medical schools and has expanded around the world and beyond medical education into a host of other disciplines. It has also galvanized the push to get students out of the lecture hall and into more interactive learning settings. This chapter is designed with two purposes in mind: to help a medical teacher decide whether to use PBL in either their course or broader medical curriculum and, having decided to use PBL, help them prepare for their role as a teacher in a PBL course. Teaching in a PBL course is a much different experience than in almost any other teaching format. As Howard Barrows, the person most closely associated with the broad adoption of PBL, liked to say, rather than "being a sage on the stage, you are a guide on the side." This takes some getting used to, particularly if you like being a sage and/or you crave the stage, or you just have never experienced a form of teaching where you were not THE authoritative source.

Definition of PBL

PBL can be characterized as an instructional method that uses patient problems as a context for students to acquire knowledge about the basic and clinical sciences. It is most commonly associated with small group learning in which the instructor serves as a facilitator. As a facilitator, the instructor's role is to ensure that the process of PBL is carried out, not to dispense knowledge. The process of PBL is to place the focus on the students and to allow them free inquiry into how to solve the problem. Specifically, the facilitator has three tasks: to help students organize their group to

M.A. Albanese (✉)
University of Wisconsin School of Medicine and Public Health, Madison, WI, USA

W.B. Jeffries, K.N. Huggett (eds.), *An Introduction to Medical Teaching*,
DOI 10.1007/978-90-481-3641-4_4, © Springer Science+Business Media B.V. 2010

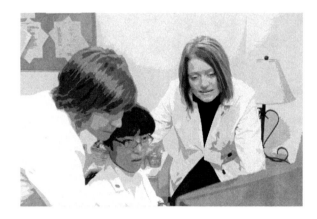

function effectively, to ensure that all members of the group have an opportunity to participate fully, and to adjust their course if they deviate too far from the desired path. Originally, PBL was designed to be an overarching curriculum that required a major reallocation of time allotted to various educational activities. After the time for structured activities was reduced, there was a major restructuring in how the remaining required time was allocated to lecture, small group, lab, etc. A number of medical schools maintain two curriculum tracks, one traditional lecture-based and the other PBL. In recent years, there has been a trend for schools that have dual tracks to merge them into one, adopting the best of both curricula into a single combined "hybrid" curriculum. There have also been efforts to institute PBL in individual courses embedded within curricula that employed largely lecture-based learning methods.

Research on the effectiveness of PBL has been somewhat disappointing to those who expected PBL to be a radical improvement in medical education. Several reviews of PBL over the past 20 years have not shown the gains in performance that many had hoped for; such studies have been limited by design weaknesses inherent in evaluating curricula. While the research indicates that PBL curricula have not produced graduates who are demonstrably inferior to graduates of other types of curricula; whether they are superior is an open question. There is some evidence that students from a PBL curriculum function better in clinically related activities and students and faculty consistently report enjoying learning and teaching in a PBL format. However, there has been concern expressed that students in a PBL curriculum may develop less complete cognitive scaffolding for basic science material. This may relate to the somewhat disconcerting trend that approximately 5–10% of students do not do well in a PBL curriculum. If able these students often change tracks after having difficulty in the PBL track. However, as schools have merged tracks into hybrid curricula, it is not clear yet how such students will do in the hybrid.

Introducing PBL into the Curriculum

The challenges likely to be encountered in implementing PBL depend to a large degree upon the scope of implementation that is being considered. If it is a change in the entire medical curriculum, it will be a much different process than if a course director is deciding whether to implement it in his/her course. In either case, a review of the evidence for and against PBL would be an important first step. The gains that are hoped for will need to be weighed against the cost to make the change. The arguments used for changing to PBL will be more compelling if they are buttressed by evidence. This will be especially important if the change is to be curriculum-wide as opposed to a single course. There were three reviews published in 1993 that have generally served this purpose. Vernon and Blake (1993) reported a meta-analysis of controlled trials, Albanese and Mitchell (1993) reported what might be considered a best evidence synthesis and Berkson (1993) conducted a thematic review. There have been more recent reports in the literature that postulate that a large degree of change should be expected from PBL to offer sufficient evidence (Colliver, 2000; Cohen, 1977). While the outcomes have not been overwhelmingly different for PBL, what may give PBL an edge over lecture-based learning is the ability to exercise greater control over the content and information density of the curriculum. Adding a lecture or making an existing lecture more dense (curriculum creep) can be done with little or no fanfare in a lecture-based curriculum. In contrast, increasing the number of problems or changing the nature of a problem to make it more information dense would demand careful consideration by PBL curriculum managers. The added scrutiny that changes demand in a PBL curriculum puts a damper on curriculum creep.

If you wish to implement PBL in your class, you should consider how to do this within the larger curriculum and the physical space and teaching constraints. Students need to have the ability to meet together in small groups with a facilitator and have access to information resources. Implementation in a course is also challenging because the types of problems that take the fullest advantage of the PBL structure tend to be multidisciplinary. The ideal situation is to have dedicated space for each small group that is equipped with technical support that allows internet access, electronic capture of white-board writing, and refreshments. However, this level of support is unlikely to be feasible in a single class use of PBL and the logistics of using multidisciplinary cases in a single course can be extremely difficult to manage. However, with some creativity and relaxing of the generally accepted requirements, it has been done (see Farrell et al., 1999).

Implementation across the entire medical school curriculum takes substantial effort. In schools that have made a major shift to PBL, the impetus or at least unquestioned support of the medical school Dean has been a driving force. There are resource allocation issues for space, faculty salary support and technical support that make any such implementation without the Dean's full support virtually impossible. Consensus among faculty is critical to begin implementation. The evidence and reviews cited earlier have been helpful to the governing bodies that have made such decisions. New medical schools have had the most success in starting PBL curricula (e.g., McMaster, Florida State University). There have been cases where whole medical school curricula have been converted to PBL, examples include the University of Iowa College of Medicine, Sherbrooke University, and the University of Missouri-Columbia. More commonly, schools have adopted a PBL track, in which admission is competitive and only a fraction of the entire class who volunteer and apply for the PBL track are admitted. Examples of this approach include Southern Illinois University, University of New Mexico, Harvard University and Michigan State University. The advantages of adopting a track approach are that it does not require a commitment from all faculty, small groups can usually be accommodated more easily, the value and feasibility of PBL can be demonstrated for those who have doubts, and all of the "bugs" in the PBL system can be worked out in a more controlled manner. In many cases, schools that began by adopting a track have eventually merged the PBL and traditional tracks into a hybrid that looks more like PBL than the traditional lecture-based learning curriculum.

Curriculum and Course Design

According to Barrows (1985), PBL is most compatible with an organ-based curriculum, in which courses are aligned with different organs of the body. Thus, a course on the cardiovascular system would have the anatomy, physiology, biochemistry, etc. of the cardiovascular system all integrated. Because patient problems are often localized to a single organ system, it seems logical that PBL would be consistent with an organ-based curriculum. For a course embedded in a lecture-based learning curriculum, those courses that are clinically focused are most compatible with a PBL format. In this type of curriculum, adopting PBL in basic science courses such as biochemistry or physiology will be more difficult due to the limited focus of the course. Integrating concepts that are the focus of other courses into the PBL cases of your course can be challenging to coordinate at the very least.

PBL Definitions

Before going into the larger issues of how to support PBL course design, it will be helpful to give a more specific definition of what has been considered the prototype PBL process (reiterative PBL in Barrow's taxonomy, 1986).

1. The process begins with a patient problem. Resources accompanying the problem include detailed objectives, print materials, audiovisual resources, multiple choice self-assessment exercises and resource faculty.
2. Students work in small groups, sometimes called tutorial groups; 6–8 students per group is often recommended.

3. The small groups are moderated by one or more faculty facilitators (sometimes called tutors, I prefer to use the term facilitator because a tutor to me is someone with content expertise that is trying to individually teach a student).
4. Students determine their own learning needs to address the problem, make assignments to each other to obtain needed information and then return to report what they have learned and continue with the problem. This happens repeatedly as students secure more information and keep probing deeper into the problem.
5. Students return for a final debriefing and analyze the approach they took after getting feedback on their case report.
6. Student evaluation occurs in a small group session and is derived from input from self, peer and facilitator.

Although Barrows' reiterative PBL is probably the purest form of what has been called PBL, there have been many different approaches used. Dolmans et al. (2005) indicate that "Although PBL differs in various schools, three characteristics can be considered as essential: problems as a stimulus for learning, tutors as facilitators and group work as stimulus for interaction" (p. 735). While the "McMaster Philosophy" had three key features: self-directed learning, problem-based learning, and small group tutorial learning, the only characteristic that is common among PBL forms is that learning is based upon patient problems.

PBL Problems

From a curriculum or course design perspective, you have to be clear about what you want to accomplish from PBL and plan accordingly. The focal points of curriculum planning are the PBL problems. The content of the problems needs to be carefully considered as well as the organization and timing.

There are 7 qualities of an appropriate problem that have been delineated:

1. Present a common problem that graduates would be expected to be able to handle, and be prototypical of that problem.
2. Be serious or potentially serious – where appropriate management might affect the outcome.
3. Have implications for prevention.
4. Provide interdisciplinary input and cover a broad content area.
5. Lead students to address the intended objectives.
6. Present an actual (concrete) task.
7. Have a degree of complexity appropriate for the students' prior knowledge (Albanese and Mitchell, 1993).

The structure or format of the problem, sometimes called a case, provides room for much variability. They can range from brief paragraphs describing a symptom or set of symptoms (e.g., chest pain) to elaborate paper or computer simulations or even using simulated patients. They can be relatively unorganized, unsynthesized, and open-ended, or they can be relatively highly structured with specific questions that need to be addressed. Barrows (1985) suggests open-ended problems, which promote application of clinical reasoning skills, structuring of knowledge in useful contexts, and development of self-directed learning. In the same curriculum, some problems can be highly structured, particularly early in the curriculum and others unstructured, especially as students approach the end of the curriculum. An example of a type of problem that is relatively structured is the Focal Problem developed at Michigan State University. It starts with a written narrative of a clinical problem as it unfolds in a real-life setting. In this design, after descriptions of significant developments occur, "stop and think" questions are inserted for students to ponder. This approach helps students focus on the steps in the decision-making process used in solving problems that may have more than one viable solution (Jones et al., 1984; Wales and Stager, 1972; Pawlak et al., 1989). These varied problem designs and computer-based variants may all have a role at some point in a PBL curriculum. More structured formats might be better placed early in the curriculum when students will be challenged with even the simplest clinical scenarios while the lesser structured formats may be more effective after students gain clinical experience and comfort with the PBL method.

In curriculum design, you have to determine whether PBL will be used just for students to learn the basic sciences or whether it will continue into what are considered the clinical years. The topics and structure of the problems need to be carefully considered and tailored to the developing competency of students. The number of problems addressed needs to be considered. If problems are addressed in weeklong blocks, then the curriculum design for PBL is a sequence of problems equal to the number of weeks in the curriculum. The flow of the problems in terms of content, objectives and level of structure then becomes the backbone of the curriculum.

Student Groups

Next to the problems, the most important component of PBL is the grouping of students to work on the problem. As noted above, small groups of 6–8 are usually recommended. If the groups are too large, less assertive students have a reduced opportunity to provide input into deliberations and it gets difficult to schedule time for group meetings.

It is probably best to assign students to groups at random and to avoid including students who are couples (dating, married or otherwise related) in the same group. To the extent possible, groups should be comparable in their range of ability similar to the range for the entire class. It has become increasingly clear that just throwing a group of students together with a problem is not necessarily going to yield something useful. Guidelines and role assignments are often recommended to help students get a start in how to organize themselves to do productive work. Barrows (1985) (see pp. 60–61) recommends that students assume three separate administrative roles to make the process work smoothly: PBL reader, Action Master List Handler, and Recorder. New students should assume these roles with each new problem.

Effective groups establish basic norms of acceptable behavior. For example, the group should determine when interruption is permitted, the attitudes towards latecomers, whether eating is allowed during a session, what to do if the tasks for the day are completed early and so on. Technology is also becoming an issue for small group management and may interfere with problem-solving in any number of ways. Computers, cell phones, PDAs, MP3 players, etc., can all be used for distracting purposes. Ground rules for the use of technology should be part of the standards of acceptable behavior (e.g., no checking email, or receiving non-emergency phone calls during the session).

Small Group Facilitator

The next major participant is the facilitator(s). Who should be a facilitator has been a somewhat controversial matter. There is some evidence that having content "expert" facilitators improves student performance, especially early in the curriculum. However, it is unrealistic to have facilitators who are expert in all areas that are the subject of PBL cases. Some schools actively avoid selecting content expert facilitators to reduce student dependence upon them as information sources. Facilitators need knowledge sufficient to achieve a level of familiarity with the material. Typically facilitators need to work through a case 3 times to achieve what has been called "case expertness" (Zeitz and Paul, 1993).

What facilitators mostly need is adequate preparation for their role. They need to be given specific guidelines for how they are to interact with students. Moving from content expert to facilitator is not necessarily a natural act for many faculty, so having them practice their role during training will be helpful. The use of "standardized" students, a group of people who are trained to act like students, can make the practice closer to the real thing. However, it can be expensive and the fidelity of the simulation to real life may be difficult to maintain.

Facilitators should also be given all information about the case and any associated readings or materials that students will be given, but in addition, materials that will

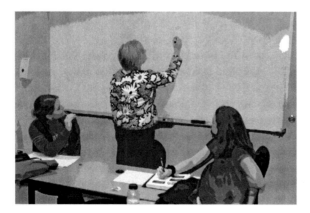

allow them to be able to guide students in their search for knowledge. This includes the "next steps" that students are expected to take. If there are preparatory lectures, it will benefit the facilitators to attend. Anything that can help facilitators function in a facilitator role and achieve case expertness is useful.

Facilitators also need to be prepared for students' reaction to the experience. If students are used to having faculty serving as content deliverers, not facilitators, the transition to this type of relationship can be rocky. Facilitators need to be prepared for student frustration early in the process when the facilitator does not give them direct answers to their questions. Over time, students learn that the facilitator is explicitly not to be a source of answers to their questions, but early on it can be a difficult adjustment for students and facilitators.

How many facilitators per group (or how many groups per facilitator) is as much a practical consideration as one that is educational. The obvious answer is at least one facilitator per group would be ideal. However, faculty resources are often quite limited. A number of schools have successfully used more advanced students as facilitators or as a co-facilitator with a faculty member. There have also been studies that examined the impact of having faculty facilitate more than one group at once, circulating between them. When the facilitator cannot be with a group throughout its deliberations, it makes it difficult for the facilitator to re-engage with the group and it takes additional time that must be factored into the process. A circulating facilitator is also limited in their ability to ensure that there is balanced input from all members of the group and assess student contributions to the group process.

In summary, the qualifications of the facilitators are probably not as important as their familiarity and comfort with the cases. How many facilitators are needed depends upon how many groups and the number of facilitators used per group and the availability of facilitators. Advanced students have been used as co-facilitators with faculty to good advantage. Using fewer than one facilitator per group has significant trade-offs in terms of the facilitator's ability to manage disruptive or dysfunctional group dynamics and to evaluate student contributions to the group process.

PBL Process

The actual process used in conducting PBL can vary, but the Maastricht 7 Step method (Wood, 2003) is often used as a guide for facilitators and students:

Step 1 – Identify and clarify unfamiliar terms presented in the scenario; scribe lists those that remain unexplained after discussion.

Step 2 – Define the problem or problems to be discussed; students may have different views on the issues, but all should be considered; scribe records a list of agreed problems.

Step 3 – "Brainstorming" session to discuss the problem(s), suggesting possible explanations on basis of prior knowledge; students draw on each other's knowledge and identify areas of incomplete knowledge; scribe records all discussion.

Step 4 – Review steps 2 and 3 and arrange explanations into tentative solutions; scribe organizes the explanations and restructures if necessary.

Step 5 – Formulate learning objectives; group reaches consensus on the learning objectives; tutor ensures learning objectives are focused, achievable, comprehensive, and appropriate.

Step 6 – Private study (all students gather information related to each learning objective).

Step 7 – Group shares results of private study (students identify their learning resources and share their results); tutor checks learning and may assess the group.

Grading Student Performance

Evaluating student performance in PBL is challenging. To treat it adequately would take a separate publication all by itself, perhaps a text. One of the difficulties in evaluating PBL is that the process used to solve a problem is often as important as the solution reached. Further, problem-solving in a facilitated small group is a complex task that involves social interactions and that unfolds sequentially over time. Capturing such skills in an assessment is difficult. For example, knowledge assessments have been used to assess students in PBL curricula, but they do not lend themselves very effectively for capturing the interactions that occurred during the small group sessions. Facilitator ratings would probably be better, but having facilitators rate student performance can affect group dynamics. And, if students are used as facilitators or co-facilitators, the situation becomes even more complex.

Two measures are heavily linked to PBL that are worth describing: Triple jump exercise and Objective Structured Clinical Exams (OSCEs).

The primary goal of a triple jump exercise is to assess clinical problem-solving and self-directed learning skills. In a triple jump exercise, students discuss a written clinical scenario and identify the related learning goals, review the learning materials individually, and return to present their conclusions and judge their own performances. Students sometimes have 3 h to complete their exercise, sometimes a week. This type of assessment is often used for formative evaluation purposes. It is less often used for grading purposes because it is time consuming and limits the number of scenarios that can be evaluated. As a result scores tend to be contextually bound to the specific problem assessed. I personally think the name choice is unfortunate because it is too close to the negative term "jumping through hoops."

Objective Structured Clinical Examinations are performance-based examinations in which students rotate from station to station (Harden et al., 1975). At each station, students are required to do a particular task or sequence of tasks (e.g., interview a patient and perform a physical exam and then write up their assessment). There are two general types of OSCE stations, the long and short type. The long type of station can take up to a couple of hours to complete and is very extensive. The short type is much more focused and stations generally take from 10 to 15 min. The Clinical Skills portion of the United States Medical Licensure Examination Step 2 is of the short type. For the first 15 years of their existence, OSCEs were not widely adopted for high stakes evaluation purposes due to a pervasive problem with what was termed content specificity. Student performance varied quite markedly when even small changes in the nature of the content of a station were made. In the late 1980s and early 1990s, a series of studies (Colliver et al., 1989; Petrusa et al., 1991) applied generalizability theory to the problem. They were able to project acceptable reliability for OSCEs for making pass–fail decisions with at least 10 stations however, reliability was found to vary dramatically between schools (Berkson, 1993; Dolmans et al., 2005) and needs to be assessed with each application. OSCEs have achieved widespread adoption since that time. Stations often use standardized patients, computer simulations, literature search facilities, manikins, and other types of "hands-on" experiences. The strengths of the OSCE are its face validity and standardized clinical experience for all examinees. There are relatively few other ways of assessing complex skills and abilities such as communication skills with the same degree of standardization and reliability. The primary limitation of the OSCE pertains to the resources needed for implementation. For an in-depth discussion of the use of OSCEs in any curriculum, see Chapter 11. For readers who are interested in a thorough treatment of assessment of students in PBL, Nendaz and Tekian (1999) provide an overview. For an analysis of the strengths and weaknesses of various approaches to student assessment, see Chapter 11.

Resources

PBL can be resource intensive depending upon how it is implemented. However, a lecture-based learning curriculum is also resource intensive. It has been estimated that for class sizes less than 100, PBL may have a cost advantage (Albanese and Mitchell, 1993). However, the costs of computing and the like have come down since then, but faculty time has generally become more expensive. With the rising cost of faculty time for serving as facilitators, the breakeven point between lecture and PBL has become less favorable to PBL.

In the early implementations of PBL, small groups were given dedicated space. Those who have dedicated space generally think it is very important for creating a sense of group cohesion and giving the group a place to meet at any time. It also helps to justify the tuition that many schools charge! However, dedicated space in today's crowded health sciences learning centers can be hard to come by and increasingly hard to justify. As schools respond to the anticipated shortage of physicians by increasing class sizes, they will be even more hard-pressed to supply dedicated space for PBL groups. While it is not hard to see how dedicated space would be a desirable feature, it is not necessarily clear that the lack of dedicated space will have detrimental effects on student learning.

What all small groups will need is access to information resources. Having dedicated space for groups enabled institutions to furnish them with secured computers that could be used for searching the literature or the web. However, with the increasing availability of notebook computers and remote access to the web, dedicated space for information access is not as critical. Students can even meet at the local coffee shop and have web access, something they may actually prefer. Generally, each group should have at least one computer available during their meetings. The computer is needed for recording the proceedings and accessing information resources. If a single person serves as the recorder and manages access to the information resources, some of the potential problems associated with abuse of technology can be minimized.

A well-stocked library is an important need for students in a PBL curriculum. Nolte et al. (1988) found that library use of reserve books increased twenty fold after introducing a PBL course on neurobiology into the curriculum. With the more recent advent of the internet and online references, having internet access is essential. Literature search software such as PubMed is critical. Having general web-searching capability is useful for looking for non-library references such as policy statements and current events. However, as noted by Kerfoot and colleagues (2005), there need to be guidelines for internet usage to avoid having the problem solving process subverted by web searches and non-authoritative sources.

Also beneficial are white-boards or blackboards. Some schools have adopted electronic blackboards that enable electronic capturing of the material students write on the board.

Lectures can also be an instructional resource, but Barrows recommends limiting them to 1–1.5 h per day (Barrows, 1985). Barrows also recommends that basic science research faculty should be a resource available to meet with students for 4–6 h per week.

With new learners, there is a danger of having too many resource options. They can bog down looking for information and give too little attention to problem-solving. The facilitator should be quick to intervene should it happen.

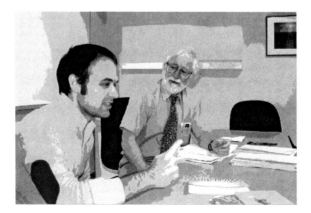

The instructional environment in the small group should be informal and as low stress as possible. Lighting should be sufficient to see all the types of educational resources that will be shared. The environment (chairs) should be comfortable, but not so comfortable as to make it difficult for students to stay alert. Students should be able to bring food and drink into the meeting room. Ready access to a refrigerator and even microwave help to make the room comfortable.

Summary

Beginning a PBL curriculum is not for the faint-hearted. There is much infrastructure that needs to be put into place and there may be increased costs. While the effectiveness of PBL appears to be gaining better documentation and we are gaining a better understanding about how to do PBL, there is still much we need to learn. In the meantime, it is important to keep in mind what one is trying to accomplish with PBL. Based upon recent learning principles, Dolmans et al. (2005) identified four important processes (constructive, self directed, collaborative and contextual) underlying PBL that provide a good synopsis of what one is trying to accomplish. By a constructive process, it is meant that learning is an active process by which students "construct or reconstruct their knowledge networks." A self-directed process is one where learners are involved in planning, monitoring and evaluating the learning process. A collaborative learning process is one in which the social structure involves two or more students interacting in which they: have a common goal, share responsibilities, are mutually dependent and need to reach agreement through open interaction. A contextual process recognizes that learning is context-bound and that transfer to different contexts requires confronting cases or problems from multiple perspectives. No matter how one decides to ultimately implement PBL, it is important that they design their experience to keep clearly in mind what they are trying to accomplish and not get distracted from their goal.

References

Albanese MA, Mitchell S (1993) Problem-based learning: A review of literature on its outcomes and implementation issues. Academic Medicine 68: 52–81.

Barrows HS (1985) How to design a problem-based curriculum for the preclinical years. Springer, New York.

Barrows HS (1986) A taxonomy of problem-based learning methods. Medical Education 20: 481–486.

Berkson L (1993) Problem-based learning. Have the expectations been met? Academic Medicine 68: S79–S88.

Cohen J (1977) Statistical power analysis for the behavioral sciences, rev ed. Englewood Cliffs, Mahwah, NJ.

Colliver J (2000) Effectiveness of problem based learning curricula. Academic Medicine 75: 259–266.

Colliver JA, Verhulst SJ, Williams R, Norcini JJ (1989) Reliability of performance on standardized patient cases: A comparison of consistency measures based on generalizability theory. Teaching and Learning in Medicine 1(1): 31–37.

Dolmans DHJM, De Grave W, Wolfhagen IHAP, van der Vleuten CPM (2005) Problem-based learning: Future challenges for educational practice and research. Medical Education 39: 732–741.

Farrell T, Albanese MA, Pomrehn P (1999) Problem-based learning in ophthalmology: A pilot program for curricular renewal. Archives of Ophthalmology 117: 1223–1226.

Harden RM, Stevenson M, Downie WW, Wilson GM (1975) Assessment of clinical competence using objective structured examination. British Medical Journal 1: 447–451.

Jones JW, Bieber LL, Echt R, Scheifley V, Ways PO (1984) A problem-based curriculum – ten years of experience. In: Schmidt HG, de Volder ML (eds) Tutorials in problem-based learning. Van Gorcum, Assen/Maastricht, Netherlands.

Kerfoot BP, Masser BA, Hafler JP (2005) Influence of new educational technology on problem-based learning at Harvard Medical School. Medical Education 39(4): 380–387.

Nendaz MR, Tekian A (1999) Assessment in problem-based learning medical schools: A literature review. Teaching and Learning in Medicine 11(4): 232–243.

Nolte J, Eller P, Ringel SP (1988) Shifting toward problem-based learning in a medical school neurobiology course. In: Research in medical education. Proceedings of the twenty-seventh annual conference. Association of American Medical Colleges, Washington, DC, pp. 66–71.

Pawlak SM, Popovich NG, Blank JW, Russell JD (1989) Development and validation of guided design scenarios for problem-solving instruction. American Journal of Pharmaceutical Education 53: 7–16.

Petrusa ER, Blackwell T, Carline J, Ramsey P, McGahie W, Colindres R, Kowlowitz V, Mast T, Soler NA (1991) A multi-institutional trial of an objective structured clinical examination. Teaching and Learning in Medicine 3: 86–94.

Vernon DTA, Blake RL (1993) Does problem-based learning work? A meta-analysis of evaluative research. Academic Medicine 68: 550–563.

Wales CE, Stager R (1972) Design of an educational system. Engineering Education 62: 456–459.

Wood DF (2003) ABC of learning and teaching in medicine: Problem based learning. British Medical Journal 326: 328–330.

Zeitz HJ, Paul H (1993) Facilitator expertise and problem-based learning in PBL and traditional curricula. Academic Medicine 68(3): 203–204.

Chapter 5
Team-Based Learning

Kathryn K. McMahon

Team-Based Learning (TBL) is a large group, peer teaching strategy, that can alternately be described as an expert-led, interactive and analytical teaching strategy. TBL keeps the class together (large group) with one or more expert(s) while the students apply the content to specific problems (analytical) in small groups (interactive) at intervals during the learning session. The students are expected to prepare prior to the session. Content is *used* throughout the session rather than simply introduced. This approach allows students to practice with the content under the watchful eye of the expert.

Larry Michaelsen originated TBL in the late 1970s at the University of Oklahoma business school. It came to the attention of medical education in the late 1990s when Boyd Richards and colleagues began piloting it at Baylor School of Medicine. Through funds from the US Department of Education this group introduced TBL to the medical education world by hosting a series of annual conferences and by presenting TBL at untold numbers of schools and professional meetings. There is now an annual conference focused on TBL that is held by the TBL Collaborative, a non-profit professional organization that evolved out of those early conferences. More information about that group and its conferences can be found at the TBL Collaborative webpage (http://tblcollaborative.org). Another very useful webpage about TBL is the Team-Based Learning webpage (http://teambasedlearning.apsc.ubc.ca). The TBL Collaborative provides consultants to help with early implementation of TBL. Information about these consultants can be found at both of the web pages given above.

A thorough discussion of TBL is given in a recent text by Michaelsen et al. (2008a). Details of TBL philosophy, along with implementation instructions, are provided in the book. The book also features several short chapters on experiences of medical faculty that might be of assistance to a first time implementer of TBL.

K.K. McMahon (✉)
Department of Medical Education, Paul L. Foster School of Medicine,
Texas Tech University Health Sciences Center, El Paso, TX, USA

W.B. Jeffries, K.N. Huggett (eds.), *An Introduction to Medical Teaching*,
DOI 10.1007/978-90-481-3641-4_5, © Springer Science+Business Media B.V. 2010

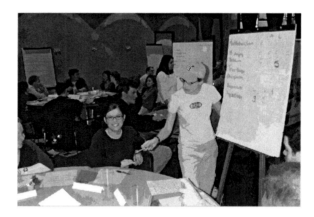

TBL Fundamentals

TBL is best used as a course strategy rather than a rarely used deviation from didactic lecture. That said, it can be used very effectively at any "dosage." Thus, TBL can be successful when used as the sole teaching method, as part of a hybrid of teaching methods or even only once in a course. The more students and faculty use it the more comfortable they are with it. With increased comfort, less time is spent on the process and more preparatory and session time is devoted to content and its application. As with most endeavors, the more time invested by the faculty, the higher the quality of experience for students. Likewise the better prepared the student comes to a TBL session the more they will get out of that session.

A TEAM Versus a Small Group

The difference between "small group" and "team" needs to be addressed as one considers the "dosage" of TBL that will be used. A team evolves out of a small group that works together for a period of time and over several sessions. TBL can also be a tool for teaching teamwork and professionalism when it is a frequently used, predominant learning method of the course. The assignment of individuals to teams is important for this use of TBL. Students' competence in some aspect(s) of the content of the course should be distributed throughout the small groups. The instructor should engineer the composition of the teams with this in mind rather than allowing students to simply self-assign themselves to groups.

It is frequently asked how long a group of students need to work together to develop into a team. As a general rule, it takes about six to eight separate sessions. Thus, from this perspective it is recommended that the groups should stay together for at least 15–20 sessions to allow students to profit from the team. Therefore, instructors commonly require that teams stay intact for one semester or an entire year.

TBL Stages

There are three stages or phases to TBL. These can all take place in and around a single session or be staggered over two or more sessions. The stages are:

a. Student Preparation.
b. Readiness Assurance.
c. Application.

Student Preparation

In the preparation stage, the student completes an assignment such as a reading, attending a lecture/session, viewing a video or performing an interview. Preparation should be guided by clear instructions/learning objectives from the instructor as to the content and depth of student understanding. The student should be given a realistic time period for this preparation. A flaw that instructors should avoid is to give an exhaustive or extensive literature/reading assignment that takes several days to read, much less understand and learn. Similarly instructors should avoid using objectives that are superficial and/or vague. For example, to assign the entire book of a leading text of renal physiology and then to give the learning objective of "Describe the normal physiology of the kidney" has two flaws. The learning objective does not give sufficient guidance to appreciate the depth and breadth of knowledge the instructor expects the student to learn. It also is unrealistic to expect a student to "consume" an entire textbook for one or even several sessions – regardless of the teaching method/strategy to be used.

Readiness Assurance

The Readiness Assurance stage uses a relatively short set of questions (e.g., quiz, exam, or test) that test understanding of key concepts found in the preparatory materials. This stage has become known as the Readiness Assurance Test (RAT). This stage has four individual steps (iRAT, gRAT, Appeals and Feedback) that revolve around allowing the individual student, small groups, and the entire group to work on content. The students individually take the test (iRAT) followed by the small groups (teams) taking the same test as groups (gRAT). To allow for student concerns that a question on the test was either ambiguous or in some other way flawed, groups are then encouraged to submit written Appeals. Finally the instructor leads a brief discussion involving all teams as a review of the test and content (Feedback). The purpose of the Readiness Assurance stage is to assure both the student and instructor that the student understands the content to the level needed for problem solving, analysis, evaluation and/or synthesis.

The RAT stage commonly takes about one hour. Recognizing that all four parts of the stage occur in that time, one can see that the nature and number of questions significantly impacts the success of this stage of TBL. New implementers of TBL often have questions about this. Commonly a multiple choice test of 10–12 questions works well. These questions should focus on the key points from the preparation materials. The questions can be layered in complexity, i.e., some are very concrete and focused on a single concept while others integrate multiple concepts. Generally assume that about 10 minutes will be used for the iRAT, 20 min for the gRAT, 5–10 min for the Appeals, and 10–15 min for the instructor Feedback.

Please note that the instructor is "teaching" only during the last 10 or so minutes. Most of the learning occurs during the first three stages of Readiness Assurance. During the iRAT, students recognize what they do not understand. During the gRAT, peer teaching occurs easily and naturally. Finally, during the Appeals, students must learn to construct a logical argument.

Usually the iRAT can be performed on an easily graded answer sheet (e.g., Scantron™). The gRAT can be completed on this same type of sheet or an Immediate Feedback-Assessment Technique (IF-AT or "scratch-off") self-scoring answer sheet. The IF-AT form allows immediate feedback to the students of each team. This serves as an additional tool for learning, commonly brings fun into the process and thus is highly recommended. This type of "scratch-off" form is available from a variety of educational supply companies and can be found by simple internet searches using the key word "IF-AT forms."

Application

The real "meat" of TBL occurs in the Application stage. Here is where students, in their teams and later in the large group discussion, really learn as they use the concepts to critically think about a situation posed to them. Application assignments are commonly a clinical or basic science experiment vignette with an accompanying question. There are a few aspects of this stage that are characteristic of TBL. Generally each application assignment has two process steps. First, the **same** assignment is given to all teams and the teams are allowed to work on the question for a time period. Second, all teams work with the instructor in the large group to evaluate and discuss the question. This happens easily by using some simple "rules" called the Four S's. The team assignment (vignette with question) should be:

(1) **Significant** to the student;
(2) The **same** for all students;
(3) Designed to make a **specific** choice; and,
(4) Reported **simultaneously** by the teams.

We will return to the Four S's in a moment but let's first talk about the time needed for a "representative" assignment in the Application stage. The Application stage can occur within the same learning session as the RAT or it can occur at one or more later sessions after the RAT is completed. The decision on which to choose is

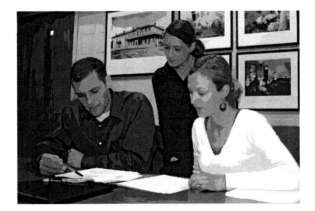

very much dependent on the nature and design of the course, the design of the learning objectives (depth and breadth) and the individual preference of the instructor. It is common that the Readiness Assurance and Application stages occur contiguously because of ease of course scheduling and other logistical issues. Thus, for a two-hour session, the first 50 min might be used for the Readiness Assurance stage and the remaining time (60–70 min) used for the Application stage. How does the instructor divide up the time within the Application stage? The concept to keep in mind is that *most* learning takes place in the team discussion of the assignment. This is when the individual students are beginning to put together the logic of the final choice. With this in mind the instructor is encouraged to allow a significant portion of time for team discussion of the assignment and a lesser portion focused on the large group discussion of team decisions. Thus if there is a 60 min block of time for the Application stage it is suggested that there be two Application assignments. For each assignment approximately 20 min should be for the individual teams to work and approximately 10 min to be used for the large group discussion. In cases where the teams are to submit a written description of their logic and choice of options, this written material should be picked up by the instructor before the large group discussion. More comments about written descriptions of Team logic are noted below.

Use of progressive cases is a "twist" that can be used to tie aspects of two assignments together. In such cases less time may be needed to review the vignette. For example a vignette might be the description of a first clinical encounter with a patient. In that vignette, clinically relevant information might be the chief complaint and physical finding. The first application might be to choose the most likely diagnosis given the physical findings from a reasonable set of differential diagnoses. That assignment might take 20 min of discussion at the team level and 10 min of large group discussion. Alternatively, the assignment might be to choose the top test that should be ordered to help develop a differential diagnosis. The next case could specifically list the result of the first assignment (top diagnosis or test performed) and a resulting question developed from that result. For example, the first assignment might ask students to choose the highest priority diagnosis. The second assignment might then reveal that the tests support a specific diagnosis and ask the team to choose the next step in the management of the patient. In this scenario the team discussion might be less intense and so only 10 min might be needed and 5–7 min for the large group discussion. Whether or not isolated assignments or progressive assignments are used, it is important to keep the Four S's in mind.

More About the Four S's

The need of *significance* of the assignment would seem obvious but it should be stressed that the *student* should be able to see that significance. Sometimes the most easily written assignment is not the most useful assignment for students. Developing a useful assignment is a very important part of TBL. Faculty often find this the most challenging part of early implementation of the TBL method/strategy. Working collaboratively or at least asking other faculty to critique the assignment is a good way to improve the quality of an application assignment.

The use of the *same* assignment for all Teams is essential for two reasons. There is a logistical reason of having a large group discussion rather than simply a collection of small group reports. To accomplish this all of the Teams must have worked on the same assignment. The second reason is that it is essential that everyone has had a chance to think about the assignment in order to encourage the maximum learning. If one student (or group of students) reports to the rest of the group on one topic (assignment) and others likewise report on other assignments, much less learning by any individual student occurs. What generally happens in this situation is that the reporter learns quite a bit about their assignment and much less about all other assignments. They are actively engaged in their assignment and most likely passively engaged in other assignments.

The rule of the assignment requiring a *specific* choice is very important to TBL. This aspect differs from other small group learning methods which commonly allow for open-ended questions that foster an open discussion between individual students and/or the instructor. The use of a specific choice fosters critical thinking by making participants choose from among various options thus, students must learn how to make decisions at the individual, team and collective session levels. This is particularly true if the options are all plausible alternatives at the level of the students' understanding. Thus, while the structure of the vignette/question appears to be very similar to a single-best answer multiple choice question, it really can go beyond that. More than one of the options might be correct. The logic the team used to select the option they chose is the core of the work. The team should be able to logically explain why they chose one option over the others including why they did not chose the other options. Some faculty who use TBL specifically ask the teams to write their logic and submit it for evaluation by the instructor. Others simply listen to the team's oral presentation of the logic at the large group step of the session. Either way, the real learning comes from the individual student thinking about and discussing with their team, the various advantages and disadvantages of the options and making a *specific* choice from those options.

The "rule" of *simultaneous reporting* of the teams' choice is also very important to TBL. Since the development of the logic of the team's choice is important to the learning within the Application stage, it is important that all teams simultaneously report which option they picked so that no team can rely on another team for the logic. Any team might be asked to defend their choice, so they must be prepared to do that at the moment of the simultaneous reporting. Simultaneous reporting is easily accomplished by giving each team a set of numbered placards that correspond to the various choices. The instructor then announces to the entire session attendees that all teams are to raise the appropriate placard at a particular time point (e.g., "on the count of three"). The instructor then recognizes the distribution of responses among teams. Then the instructor can initiate a discussion by asking randomly one team to state one point that they considered in their decision. Rather than allowing that team to give all points in their decision, the instructor can shift to another team and ask them to respond to that point and to add one point from their team's discussion. Thus the instructor can orchestrate the discussion, occasionally ask a team why they did not consider one of the options the team did not pick, bring up an unaddressed concept that is important, or praise the logic used by all or particular teams.

Essential TBL Principles

TBL has some essential components. These make TBL unique from other learning strategies.

Team Formation and Maintenance

Team formation is critical. Resources students bring to the class should be distributed evenly throughout the teams. For example, in a pharmacology course, those students who have previously worked in a pharmacy might have a wealth of knowledge about medications and their use. Thus, those individuals should be assigned to different teams to prevent the concentration of pharmacologic knowledge on one team. The instructor should consider what knowledge base would best be distributed throughout the Teams. Tips about methods to do this easily can be found at the Team-Based Learning webpage (http://teambasedlearning.apsc.ubc.ca) and in several of the texts written for using TBL (Michaelsen et al., 2004; Michaelsen et al., 2008a, b).

Team maintenance is another issue that must be considered if TBL is being used as a predominant teaching method in a course. Some Teams or individuals in a given Team can be dysfunctional and cause disruption to either the Team or the class. Instructors should understand that the Team building process goes through normal group dynamics phases (sometimes referred to as forming, storming, norming and performing). This process may make "bumps in the road" for some Teams but normally will work themselves out without intervention by the instructor. Scheduling some time for training the class about the TBL process and peer assessment helps with normal team maintenance. Open discussions or feedback sessions about how things are going and instructors' willingness to listen to student concerns often will help ease tensions. In extreme cases, changing the team composition might be needed but only as a last resort.

Student Accountability and Incentive

A second essential component of TBL is that all students are accountable. Students learn best when there is an immediate need and an appropriate incentive. Grading performance can be used to hold students accountable for their learning in TBL and thereby evaluation of performance is an immediate incentive. TBL is designed so that the individual student is held accountable for their acquisition of knowledge if the iRAT is graded. Also the individual's ability to use the knowledge and cooperate with other team members are accountable if the gRAT and Application assignments are graded. As the small groups develop into teams, the individual members learn what attribute each team member brings to the group and learn to use those attributes to make the team most successful. Thus gRATs and applications are also evidence of each team member's knowledge. Thus, each TBL session provides several opportunities for students to be held accountable. Of course, the ability to work in the team and the development of professionalism are other very important aspects of TBL for which students can be accountable.

TBL can and should include the evaluation of each team member by their team peers for helpfulness and professionalism. This aspect of the evaluation should not be done at each session but should be done only occasionally, such as at a midpoint and at the end of the course. Peer evaluation can be done by a relatively short list of specific questions to which the students respond for each of their peers. The instructor must help the students understand the importance of peer evaluation. This is best done by frank discussion with the students as to the frequency of use, and the need for honest constructive criticism. The instructor should demonstrate how to give and receive such constructive evaluation. The Team-Based Learning webpage (http://teambasedlearning.apsc.ubc.ca) gives useful tips about Peer Evaluation.

Real-Time Feedback

TBL also provides an opportunity to give frequent feedback in real time. This occurs in the Readiness Assurance stage by immediate scoring of the iRAT and/or the use of IF-AT answer sheets. If neither of these tools can be used, the instructor can distribute answer placards as described previously for Application assignments. Electronic audience response systems could also be used to identify team choices for the questions. By any of these routes the instructor can give feedback at the time the students are most acutely aware of their thought processes. This is an important component of the learning and consolidation of knowledge process. Frequent feedback is most useful to reinforce student learning when it addresses small increments of the overall learning objectives.

Similarly, the Application stage allows students to gain feedback from their peers and from the instructor as they develop and use their knowledge base to develop their logic of arguments. Corrections can be made as the logic is developed and as the student gains expertise in using their knowledge. This can be reinforced by the instructor's praise and encouragement.

Team Development and Peer-Teaching

Finally, team assignments in the Application stage must promote both learning and team development. These assignments must truly require use of the learning content but also require group interaction. Peer education is a significant aspect of TBL. The essence of TBL is lost if the assignment simply can be broken up into small components and the individual students cover different aspects. It is the peer education that drives team formation. Because of the development of teams, TBL can be used to teach professionalism. Good teams work well together because the members trust and respect each other, contribute consistently and can be relied upon.

Proof of Usefulness of TBL for Student Success and Student Satisfaction

There is a growing bibliography of research on TBL implementation (Levine et al., 2004; Meeuwsen and Pedersen, 2006; Searle et al., 2003; Thompson et al., 2007), its usefulness in learning (McInerney, 2003) and student satisfaction (Parmelee et al., 2009). A comprehensive listing of this literature is found at the Team-Based Learning webpage (http://teambasedlearning.apsc.ubc.ca/) and in the list of references below.

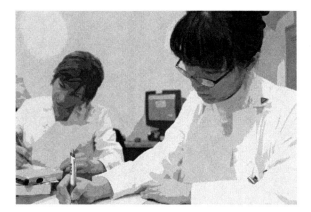

References

Levine RE, Haidet P, Lynn DJ, Stone JJ, Wolf DV, Paniagua FA (2004) Transforming a clinical clerkship with team learning. Teaching and Learning in Medicine 16(3): 270–275.

McInerney MJ (2003) Team-based learning enhances long-term retention and critical thinking in an undergraduate microbial physiology course. Microbiology Education Journal 4(1): 3–12.

Meeuwsen HJ, Pedersen R (2006) Group cohesion in team-based learning. Mountain Rise 3(1) (at http://mountainrise.wcu.edu).

Michaelsen, LK, Knight AB, Fink LD (Eds) (2004) Team-based learning: A transformative use of small groups in college teaching. Stylus Publishing, Sterling, VA.

Michaelsen LK, Parmelee DX, McMahon KK, Levine RE (Eds.) (2008a) Team-based learning for health professions education: A guide to using small groups for improving learning. Stylus Publishing, Sterling, VA.

Michaelsen LK, Sweet M, Parmelee DX (2008b) Team-based learning: small group learning's next big step. New Directions for Teaching and Learning 2008(116): 1–128.

Parmelee DX, DeStephen D, Borges NJ (2009) Medical students' attitudes about team-based learning in a pre-clinical curriculum. Medical Education Online 14(1) (at http://www.med-ed-online.org).

Searle NS, Haidet P, Kelly PA, Schneider V, Seidel CL, Richards BF (2003) Team learning in medical education: initial experiences at 10 institutions. Academic Medicine 78(10): S55–S58.

Thompson BM, Schneider VF, Haidet P, Levine RE, McMahon KK, Perkowski LC, Richards BF (2007) Team-based learning at ten medical schools: two years later. Medical Education 41(3): 250–257.

Web Pages

The Team-Based Learning Collaborative: http://tblcollaborative.org
Team-Based Learning: http://teambasedlearning.apsc.ubc.ca

Chapter 6
Teaching Clinical Skills

Janet M. Riddle

Being a clinician-teacher is exciting and stimulating. Most clinician-teachers simply enjoy teaching and value contributing to the development of young professionals. Clinicians also find that teaching keeps their knowledge and skills up to date. Clinical teachers are asked to fulfill a variety of roles. These include:

- Serving as a physician role model – exemplifying competent professional care of patients.
- Teaching and reinforcing clinical skills.
- Being a supervisor – providing opportunities for students to practice clinical skills with patients.
- Observing and providing feedback on student performance.
- Assisting students in linking basic sciences with clinical correlations.
- Mentoring students and facilitating their career development.

Learning teaching skills, including how to prepare for teaching and how to reflect on clinical experiences, will increase your satisfaction with teaching. Teaching in clinical settings is characterized by diversity. You may be asked to teach learners at different levels of training – from first-year medical students to resident physicians. You may also teach pharmacy students, nursing students or a multidisciplinary team of learners. I will use the word "student" throughout this chapter to refer to any of the learners you teach. Clinical teaching occurs in a variety of settings – in outpatient clinics, hospital wards, the emergency department, in the operating room, and during home visits. Any setting in which you care for patients is an opportunity for you to teach clinical skills. Although your teaching will be influenced by the kinds of patients you typically see and by the level of students you teach, the skills presented in this chapter can be used in any setting and with any of these learners.

In the following sections, we will explore each of the key phases of teaching in clinical settings: planning for teaching, teaching during the clinical encounter, and reflecting on the clinical experience.

J.M. Riddle (✉)
Department of Medical Education, University of Illinois-Chicago, College of Medicine, Chicago, IL, USA

W.B. Jeffries, K.N. Huggett (eds.), *An Introduction to Medical Teaching*,
DOI 10.1007/978-90-481-3641-4_6, © Springer Science+Business Media B.V. 2010

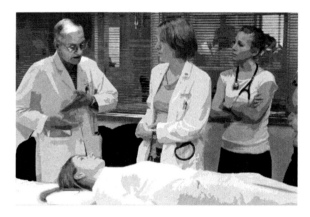

Planning for Teaching Clinical Skills

As you plan for clinical teaching, you need to understand the goals and objectives that the course or clerkship director has for the experience in which you are teaching. What are students expected to know or to be able to do as a result of your teaching? It will help you to know how the course or clerkship that you are teaching in relates to other courses and clinical experiences in the curriculum. Clinical experiences early in medical training allow students to correlate the basic sciences they are learning in the classroom with clinical problems. Later in training, students need patient care experiences to refine clinical skills and develop their fund of knowledge. You will want to plan learning activities that assist students in integrating content among courses, build on previous clinical experiences, and enhance the student's clinical capabilities.

When planning for clinical teaching, you need to consider the level of training of the student you will be working with and that student's interests and learning needs. Students early in their training are learning basic skills in interviewing and examining patients. They need opportunities both to observe you demonstrating these skills as well as opportunities to practice them with patients. Junior students are also socializing to the role of being a physician. You will want to explicitly role model professional behaviors. Students welcome mentoring that focuses on their development as novice clinicians. More advanced students are eager to refine their physical diagnosis skills. They are also developing clinical reasoning skills and capabilities in negotiating management plans with patients. Senior students are often exploring career options and are eager for your advice. Even within these generalizations, there are individual differences. You should plan to discuss goals and learning needs with each student.

Orienting Students to Facilitate Clinical Teaching

Orienting the student to your clinical setting is an important step in planning for clinical teaching. An orientation eases the student's transition to working with you and your patients. During the orientation, be sure to explain your routines in patient care. Also introduce the student to anyone else you work with, for instance nursing staff, office staff or pharmacists.

Consider what the student might learn from each of these people. Medical assistants can teach students to measure blood pressure or blood glucose. Pharmacists can teach students about medication counseling. Students value diverse experiences in clinical settings and appreciate the importance of learning to work on a healthcare team.

During the orientation, describe to the student how you provide clinical supervision and teaching. This is a key step in establishing a positive learning climate. Students appreciate clinical teachers who are enthusiastic about teaching, who inspire confidence in students' knowledge and skills, who provide feedback, and who encourage students to accept responsibility for patient care. Being enthusiastic about teaching is demonstrated by asking students about themselves and their learning needs. Students welcome your efforts to provide them with clinical experiences that are relevant to their learning needs and their stage of development. Describe for the student how clinical encounters will occur. Should the student expect to "shadow" you for some encounters? How will you observe the student's clinical skills? What information do you want included in case presentations? What kinds of notes do you expect the student to write? What teaching methods do you plan to use? Will you give assignments to the student? When and how will the student's final evaluation take place?

Don't forget to find out what the student expects to learn by working with you. Some clinical teachers use "learning contracts" to negotiate goals and expectations with the student. These contracts can include self-assessments of clinical skills, a statement of the student's goals for the experience, and planned strategies for meeting those goals. While exploring the student's expectations, you can confirm that the student understands the goals and objectives for the experience, and that you understand the other courses and clinical experiences that the student has had. Discussing the student's career interests is also helpful (Table 6.1).

Table 6.1 Keys for an effective student orientation

Review the learning goals and expectations for the clinical experience.
- Orient the student to your clinical site, patient care routines, and staff.
- Discuss your student's expectations for the experience.
- Explain your expectations of the student.
- Describe how you provide clinical supervision and teaching, including how feedback and evaluation will occur.

Selecting Patients for Clinical Teaching

You need to plan for each of the student's clinical encounters. Although teachable moments occur with every patient, you want to have a clear purpose for each clinical encounter that the student has. What will the student learn by working with this patient? Patients who have typical presentations of common diseases or prototypical clinical findings are good choices for students. Some clinical teachers select a general problem or theme for each session with a student. Students are able to observe a spectrum of patients with a similar diagnosis. Alternatively, by focusing on a clinical problem, students are able to compare and contrast different diagnoses with similar presentations. This assists students in developing concepts of the key features of diagnoses.

Plan to cover enough material with each patient encounter to stimulate the student's clinical thinking, but without overwhelming the student. Have one or two important teaching points for each encounter. The teaching points that you have selected should help the student meet the learning objectives for the clinical experience. Make sure that you have selected patients of manageable complexity for the student. At the beginning of each session, review the list of patients you are scheduled to see. Together you can select patients and discuss the teaching points that you have in mind.

Select patients who have good communication skills and who are willing to work with students. Many patients appreciate the extra attention that students give them. Patients understand the importance of teaching students. They know that they are contributing to the development of the next generation of physicians. Be sure to brief each patient about the "teaching encounter." Introduce the student, explain how the encounter will occur, solicit the patient's consent, and inform the patient that you will return after the student has finished the encounter. Respect your patient's decision to not to work with your student. Many clinical teachers find that modeling the kind of relationship that they would like students to have with patients is beneficial. A useful rule of thumb is to treat your students as you would like them to treat your patients.

Teaching During the Clinical Encounter

As a clinical teacher you will be best served by having a variety of teaching methods to use in different situations and with different learners. What is most important is that you allow students to practice skills and work with problems that will help them gain clinical competence. Let the students practice what you want them to be able to do!

Using Questions and Feedback to Enhance Clinical Reasoning

Questions play a key role in any clinical teaching. Questions stimulate and engage students; help you to determine your student's knowledge level and learning needs; and help you monitor how your students are progressing. The questions you ask can promote higher-order thinking and encourage reflection. The questions you

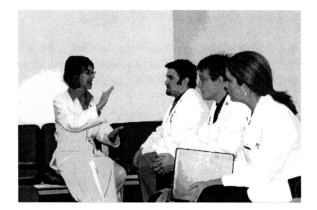

have asked, and the student's responses, are also the basis for giving constructive feedback.

When discussing clinical cases, your questions can have three purposes – to obtain factual information, to explore the student's reasoning processes, or to explore the student's learning needs. A common problem with case discussions is that questions are limited to obtaining factual information. These lower-order questions ask for more information about the patient or about what the student knows. Students may also be asked to repeat or recall what they have learned. Lower-order questions may help the clinician to care for the patient, but these questions do not help students develop clinical judgment or problem-solving skills. In contrast, you can ask questions that explore the student's understanding of the patient's clinical problem – by asking the student to formulate the problem or to think through the problem. You can also probe the uncertainties or difficulties that the student is having; thereby eliciting the student's learning needs. Exploring clinical thinking and learning needs requires higher-order questions – questions that ask students to summarize, analyze, compare and contrast, and justify. Higher-order questions also tend to be open-ended, and thus have a range of possible responses (Table 6.2).

Table 6.2 Keys to asking effective questions

- Ask one question at a time.
  - o If you ask more than one question, you increase the complexity of the learning task.
- Wait 3 s before and after the student answers.
  - o Give students time to organize their thoughts.
- Stay neutral until after the student has explained the answer.
  - o Avoid the "rapid reward" that terminates thinking.
- Use higher-order, open-ended questions.
- Create a safe environment that permits students to answer incorrectly or to guess.

The METRC Model for Case-Based Teaching

I will present two models of case-based teaching. The first is the "METRC" model, a variation of the "one-minute preceptor" or "microskills" model for teaching during clinical encounters. The steps of the "METRC" model are:

- Make a commitment.
- Explore or explain reasoning.
- Teach to the gaps.
- Reinforce what was done well.
- Correct mistakes.

After presenting a patient case to you, the student may pause or ask a question. This is your cue to ask the student to make a commitment to what she is thinking at this point. Your question allows the student to process information collected during the encounter. You are asking the student to formulate the clinical problem and to demonstrate her knowledge related to that clinical problem. Depending upon the specifics of the clinical case, your question might be "What do you think is going on with this patient?", "What is the most likely diagnosis?", "What tests would be most useful?", or "What treatment plan would you propose?" You may be tempted to ask for more factual information about the patient, but wait.

Once the student has committed to a specific diagnosis (or diagnostic strategy or treatment plan), your next question is to ask the student to explain her answer. You might ask, "What information in the history and physical led you to that diagnosis?", "What do you expect to find from the tests that you propose?", "Why did you select that medication for treating the patient, given the options available?" These questions ask students to analyze information and to justify their decisions. Two questions that are helpful to probe the student's thinking are to ask "What if the patient had …? How would that change your thinking?" and "How are … and … similar or different?" Questions that explore the student's reasoning provide opportunities for the student to reveal additional information obtained from the patient that was omitted from the original case presentation. If you still have not heard important factual information, now is the time to ask.

After hearing the student responses to the first two steps, you know where the student's gaps in knowledge or misconceptions are. The third step in the METRC model is to teach to the gaps. In general you should teach one or two important points – but not everything that you know about the patient or the diagnosis. Your teaching should match the learning needs of the student and should develop the student's knowledge and skills. The first three steps in the METRC model may be used for a brief teaching encounter or may be repeated during a more in-depth case discussion. Your student may raise questions, which you may want to assign to the student for self-directed learning.

Each clinical encounter is an opportunity to give formative feedback to the student. The final two steps in the METRC model prompt you to do so. Begin by reinforcing what the student did well. You should describe clearly the specific desirable behaviors you observed. Then correct any mistakes you observed or make suggestions for improvement. Again, you will need to be clear and specific. I will discuss feedback in more detail later in this chapter. The important point here is that you are able to give feedback based upon the student's knowledge and skills that you have probed through the questions that you have asked.

Teaching the Student to "Prime the Preceptor"

The second model for case-based teaching, SNAPPS, is an alternative to the METRC model. In this model, the student guides the clinical teaching encounter. In SNAPPS, the student primes the clinical teacher with what he needs to know or learn from the preceptor.

The student uses the following steps in clinical case presentations:

- Summarize briefly the patient's history and physical.
- Narrow the differential diagnosis to the two or three most relevant possibilities.
- Analyze the differential diagnosis by comparing and contrasting the diagnoses.
- Probe the clinical teacher by asking questions about areas of confusion, uncertainty or knowledge deficits.
- Plan management of the patient's medical issues.
- Select a focused, patient-related question for self-directed learning.

Students need to be taught this approach to case presentations. SNAPPS is a learner-centered model that focuses on both exploring the student's clinical reasoning and learning needs.

Teaching in the Patient's Presence

Teaching in the patient's presence involves a learning triad – the patient, the student, and you, the clinical teacher. Your task is to diagnose the patient's clinical problem along with the learner's abilities and needs. As discussed earlier in this chapter, it is important to prepare patients for their role in clinical teaching.

Maintaining good communication with patients during teaching encounters involves obtaining their consent, ensuring their understanding of the discussion, and allowing them to ask questions and give feedback to both you and the student. When discussing clinical information in the patient's presence, be sure to use language that the patient can understand.

As with any clinical teaching, you should have a focused purpose for teaching in the patient's presence. Using the technique of "priming" can help the student. Although priming can be used with any clinical encounter, it is especially helpful when you want to limit the time that the student spends with the patient. Simply, you identify the tasks that the student is expected to complete while with the patient and the time frame for completing the tasks. You will also want to explain what the

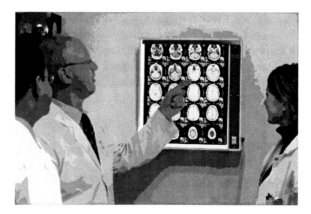

student will have accomplished as a result of the encounter, for instance a problem-focused note or an oral presentation.

Teaching Through "Active Observation"

Demonstration plays an important part in clinical teaching. In demonstrations, you ask the student to "Watch me take care of this patient." Rather than simply having students passively observe your interactions with patients, use the technique of "active observation." In this teaching method, begin by identifying what the student should learn from observing your interaction with a patient. You can use active observation with less experienced students to role model communication skills, clinical skills – including interviewing and physical examination, and professionalism. This method can also be used in complex or difficult situations, in which the student may not have the necessary knowledge or skills. Demonstrating communication skills in giving bad news to patients is an example. After identifying the learning objective, tell the student what she should do during the encounter – What should the student pay attention to? Be sure to prepare the student for whether you will ask questions or have the student repeat parts of the physical examination. After the clinical encounter, discuss what the student observed and learned from watching you.

As an example, you have a patient who is being prepared for hospital discharge. You would like your student to observe how you counsel your patient about the medications she is being discharged on. You ask your student to pay attention to how you ask your patient to repeat the instructions you have given to make sure that she understands. After asking for the student's observations, you might continue the discussion with, "How else could we have confirmed that the patient understood the discharge instructions?"

The "Two-Minute Observation"

In addition to the opportunities for role modeling, teaching in the patient's presence allows you to observe your student's clinical skills. Students are rarely observed actually interacting with patients and families. Valuable opportunities for feedback are thus missed. Observations need not be detailed or time consuming. In fact it is probably better to make multiple short observations of your student. In the "two-minute observation" the clinical teacher observes the student interacting with the patient for 2 min. The teacher and student begin by establishing the objective for the observation. You may choose to focus on how the student begins the patient interview and whether the student uses open-ended questions to explore the patient's concerns. Or you may focus on how the student counsels the patient on medications or lifestyle modification. No matter what your objective is, you will need to explain to the patient that you are observing the student and that you will return. You then make your observations and leave without disturbing the student-patient interaction. The student is now able to complete the patient visit. After the clinical encounter has concluded, give your student feedback on your observations.

Special Considerations for Teaching Physical Examination Skills

Students must perform four steps in order to make a correct diagnosis on the basis of the physical examination. Students need to anticipate the physical exam findings, perform the maneuvers necessary to elicit the findings, describe the findings that are present, and interpret the findings. In the first step, the student needs to anticipate what physical exam findings to look for based upon the patient's clinical presentation. We know that exam findings are missed because students did not think to look for them. When teaching physical examination, ask students what key findings they would expect based on the two or three most likely diagnoses explaining the patient's symptoms. The second step is to correctly perform the physical examination maneuvers that are needed to elicit the physical findings. Demonstration of correct techniques, followed by observation of the student's performance, with feedback, are important teaching techniques. For complex skills, such as hearing heart murmurs, you may need to focus on only parts of the exam, for instance, "Listen in this area. Pay attention to what you hear between the first and second heart sounds."

In the third step, the student must be able to describe the exam findings. Asking students to draw a picture of what they observed or to tap out a rhythm of what they heard can be helpful techniques to elicit their description of findings. You can help students learn the technical terms used to describe exam findings. Finally, the student interprets the exam findings in the context of the patient's history. As a clinical teacher, you should emphasize each of these four steps through asking questions, demonstrating correct techniques, and providing feedback.

Special Considerations for Teaching Procedural Skills

You can use a four-step approach to teaching procedures. This approach can be used to teach relatively simple procedures such as peripheral intravenous catheter insertion, phlebotomy, or obtaining an electrocardiogram. These steps can also be used to teach other "procedures" such as physical examination skills. This approach allows students to learn both the cognitive and psychomotor steps in performing a procedure. Even with this approach, a student may not be able to completely master a procedure if there are not sufficient opportunities for practice and feedback.

Involving the patient in teaching procedures is crucial. You must explain the student's role and your role in performing the procedure. It is your responsibility to obtain informed consent from the patient. You need to explain to the patient what is occurring while teaching or supervising the procedure.

In the first step, break down the procedure into its component parts. This includes more than the individual steps in correctly performing the procedure. It also includes the indications and contraindications for the procedure, as well as proper preparation and positioning of the patient, and use of the equipment. Demonstrate the procedure to the student in the second step. Perform your demonstration slowly – talking through each step. In the third step, you will perform the procedure, but the student will talk through each part of the procedure. These two steps allow the student to internalize the correct steps – without having to perform the motor skills necessary to complete the procedure.

The final step has the student actually perform the procedure, talking through each step that he is taking. This allows the student to add the motor skill component to the cognitive component. Depending upon the complexity of the procedure, it is clear that some procedures are best taught and learned on models or simulators. A clinical skills lab allows practice, repetition and feedback in a high-fidelity, low risk environment (see Chapter 7).

The "Final" Step in Clinical Teaching – Giving Constructive Feedback

Feedback is crucial to learning. Feedback allows students to learn about their current levels of competence and allows them to reflect on their strengths and weaknesses. Through feedback, students engage in a dialogue with a clinical teacher in order to become more competent. Feedback is the information that is given to the student that is intended to guide that student's performance. Feedback should be given regularly. As suggested by the METRC model, there are opportunities for feedback in every teaching encounter.

Constructive feedback is timely, direct and clear. Don't wait until too long after an event to give feedback. Your student will be more likely to accept your feedback and make changes, if you give feedback in a timely fashion. Be sensitive to the setting. Public areas are not conducive to well-received feedback – even if nothing "negative" is said. Students are not always aware that you are giving feedback, so start by saying, "Let me give you some feedback." Establish a positive tone. Asking your student how the rotation is going is a good way to decrease some of the student's anxiety. Then ask the student to assess her performance by describing her perceptions of strengths and areas for improvement.

Feedback should deal with specific performances that you have observed. Too often we offer generalizations such as, "Good job!" Such feedback is uninformative. You should describe the specific behaviors that you observed and the consequences of those behaviors. Be constructive – focus on what the student can do differently in a similar situation. Feedback should be based upon the goals and expectations for the clinical experience that you established during your orientation with the student.

Feedback is not evaluation. Evaluation is the summative process that occurs at the end of a course, rotation or clerkship. Even though you included feedback in every teaching encounter, you should also plan for a mid-rotation feedback session to review the student's overall performance. You may find it helpful to use the end-of-rotation evaluation form during this session. Plan to discuss to what extent the student is meeting the objectives of the experience, what competencies the students has demonstrated, and which skills need more work. Students are typically concerned about the final evaluation or grade. In these sessions, you can discuss how the student is progressing and set goals for the remainder of the rotation (Table 6.3).

Table 6.3 Keys to giving constructive feedback

- Make sure that feedback is well-timed and expected.
- Ask for the student's assessment of her performance.
- Deal with specific behaviors that you have observed.
- Don't give too much feedback at one time. Instead, give feedback regularly.
- Offer specific suggestions for improvement. Limit feedback to remediable behaviors.

The Third Phase of Clinical Teaching – Reflecting on Clinical Experiences

Reflection is important in the learning process. Reflection on clinical experiences allows students to formulate and refine clinical concepts. The process of reflection creates additional opportunities for constructive feedback. Through reflection, students plan for and anticipate what they will do in future clinical encounters. Thus reflection prepares students for future learning.

Two specific strategies for reflection include "wrap-up rounds" and homework. During wrap-up rounds, the clinical teacher and student review the patients seen during the session. Ask the student to summarize the two or three most important points from the session. A useful question to ask is, "What did you learn today that was new for you?" Other tasks that require the student to synthesize knowledge are making charts or diagrams that explain what the student understands about the

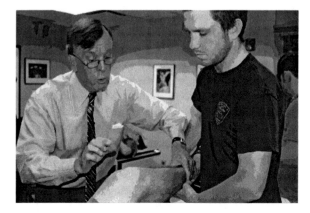

pathophysiology of the patient's clinical problem or outline the student's approach to evaluating that problem. Ask your student how he would explain the concepts learned during the session to his peers. It is also useful to ask the student to make connections between clinical experiences and classroom learning. Ask, "What are you learning in your classes that related to patients you saw today?"

Giving homework assignments is another useful reflection exercise. Reading assignments encourage self-directed, independent learning. Have your students write down the questions that they have about patients in a small notebook or on file cards. Encourage them to make the question as specific as possible. The student should select one question that she decides is most important to taking care of the patient, or most intriguing, to read about after each session. You may need to provide the student some guidance on where to look for the answer. Have the student prepare a brief summary of what was learned from the reading assignment. Don't forget to review the homework assignments with your student. Occasionally students need guidance from the clinical preceptor about choosing an appropriate question. For more advanced students, homework assignments become opportunities to build skills in evidence-based medicine.

Summary

In this chapter, you have been introduced to teaching skills related to each of the key phases of teaching in clinical settings: planning for teaching, teaching during the clinical encounter, and reflecting on the clinical experience. Discuss the goals and expectations of the rotation – and the objective of each clinical encounter – with your student. Use effective questioning skills to promote your student's clinical judgment and problem solving skills. Explicitly demonstrate communication skills, clinical skills, and professional behaviors. Make frequent observations of your student's performance in each of these areas. Give regular constructive feedback. Spend time with your student reflecting on his clinical experiences. Enjoy the satisfaction of teaching students and contributing to their professional development.

For Further Reading

Alguire PC, Dewitt DE, Pinsky LE, Ferenchick GS (2001) Teaching in your office: A guide to instructing medical students and residents. American College of Physicians Philadelphia, Philadelphia, PA.

Although written for clinicians who teach in outpatient settings, the authors offer teaching recommendations that can be adapted to any patient care setting. The "quick tips" and "tools" for preceptors are especially helpful.

Bowen JL (2006) Educational strategies to promote clinical diagnostic reasoning. New England Journal of Medicine 355: 2217–2225.

A concise review of research in the clinical diagnostic reasoning process and recommendations for clinical teachers.

Neher JO, Gordon KC, Meyer B, Stevens N (1992) A five-step "microskills" model of clinical teaching. Journal of the American Board of Family Practice 5: 419–424

This paper describes the "one-minute preceptor" or METRC model of clinical precepting.

Sachdeva AK (1996) Use of effective feedback to facilitate adult learning. Journal of Cancer Education 11: 106–118

A comprehensive review of principles and strategies for giving effective feedback.

Wolpaw TM, Wolpaw DR, Papp KK (2003) SNAPPS: A learner-centered model for outpatient education. Academic Medicine 78: 893–898

Description of a learner-centered model for case presentation that condenses the reporting of facts and encourages expression of student's thinking and reasoning.

Yudkowsky R, Otaki J, Lowenstein T, Riddle J, Nishigori H, Bordage G (2009) A hypothesis-driven physical examination learning and assessment procedure for medical students: initial validity evidence. Medical Education. 43: 729–740.

This model for teaching physical examination skills emphasizes the importance of anticipating physical findings in the context of a differential diagnosis.

Chapter 7
Teaching with Simulation

Susan J. Pasquale

The role of simulation in medical education continues to expand. It is used across the spectrum of medical education, including in medical school curricula, residency education and fellowship programs, and can be used in all health care disciplines. Applying and integrating our working knowledge of pedagogy, medical education, and medical simulation is important to both the educational and patient care missions of medical schools. Used effectively, simulation provides an environment for experiential learning toward enhancing the learner's critical thinking, problem solving, and decision-making skills. It provides opportunities to assimilate the basic and clinical sciences and to apply that knowledge in realistic, yet low risk situations. It can also improve teamwork skills and reflection.

This chapter will present information on how simulation can be optimally used to enhance the teaching and learning experience in medical education curricula. Moreover, it will offer perspectives on how simulation can re-energize teaching and learning.

What Is Simulation?

This chapter will define simulation as "a training and feedback method in which learners practice tasks and processes in life-like [face-to-face] circumstances, with feedback from observers [and] peers...to assist improvement in skills"; it is an interactive approach to teaching and learning which provides experiences that reproduce real situations (Gaba, 2004, p. i2). Simulation offers opportunities to observe learners' performance in a realistic but risk-free, controlled environment.

What Are Medical Simulators?

A "simulator" is a device that represents "a simulated patient (or part of a patient) and interacts appropriately with the actions taken by the [learner]" (Gaba, 2004,

S.J. Pasquale (✉)
University of Massachusetts Medical School, Worcester, MA, USA

W.B. Jeffries, K.N. Huggett (eds.), *An Introduction to Medical Teaching*,
DOI 10.1007/978-90-481-3641-4_7, © Springer Science+Business Media B.V. 2010

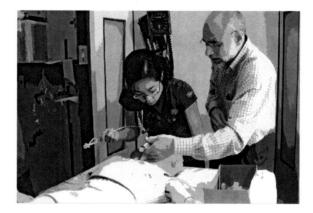

p. i2). Simulators vary from relatively simple multimedia, to various types of task trainers, to human patient simulators. Though medical simulation represents a range of technologies, the term "simulator" is generally used to refer to technologies that are used to imitate tasks. Simulators permit learners to practice procedures as often as required to reach proficiency without harm to a patient. A task trainer is a device that replicates limited aspects of a task. Though this chapter will not go into currently used simulation technologies that support teaching and learning in medical education, a snapshot of simulation technology is provided in Table 7.1 (Ziv et al., 2003, p. 784).

Table 7.1 Simulation tools and approaches used in simulation-based medical education

Tools or approach	Description
Low-tech simulators	Models or mannequins used to practice simple physical maneuvers or procedures
Simulated/standardized patients	Actors trained to role-play patients, for training and assessment of history taking physicals, and communication skills
Screens-based computer simulators	Programs to train and assess clinical knowledge and decision making, e.g., preoperative critical incident management, problem-based learning, physical diagnosis in cardiology, acute cardiology, acute cardiac life support
Complex task trainers	High-fidelity visual, audio, touch cues and actual tools that are integrated with computers. Virtual reality devices and simulators that replicate a clinical setting, e.g., ultrasound, bronchoscopy, cardiology, laparoscopic, surgery, arthroscopy, sigmoidoscopy, dentistry.
Realistic patient simulators	Computer-driven, full-length mannequins. Simulated anatomy and physiology that allow handling of complex and high risk settings, including team training and integration of multiple simulation devices.

Why Teach with Simulation: The Benefits

Learning is facilitated through experience (Kolb, 1984), and simulation has the potential to provide that experience and learning if used in keeping with basic principles of educational theory.

Simulation provides an effective vehicle for the integration of the basic and clinical sciences, and can be effectively used in curricula across the continuum of medical education and practice to make the curricular material come to life. Medical students cite critical thinking, as facilitated by experiential learning, as an important benefit of learning through simulation.

Simulation has been shown to improve the acquisition and retention of new knowledge compared with traditional lectures. Participants in the 2005 Millennium Conference on Medical Simulation agreed that "simulation offers a conducive environment for focused reflection and critical thought" (Huang et al., 2007, p. 88). The Conference report concluded that "medical simulation represents a powerful technique that has the potential to revolutionize medical education ... and to enhance current curriculum by integrating basic and complex concepts [through] reflective practice" (Huang et al., 2007, p. 93). It further reported that simulation should be used to enhance currently used methods of medical education. Gordon et al. (2001, p. 472), noted that students "felt that the [simulation] experience promoted critical thinking and active learning, and that it allowed them to build confidence and practice skills in a supportive environment." Those same students believed that the simulator helped them integrate basic and clinical sciences toward preparing for residency.

Key Principles for Teaching and Learning with Simulation

Teaching

As with any teaching effort, teaching with simulation needs to begin with an analysis of what the learners need instead of what the technology can offer. Curricula and use of simulation based on the level and needs of the learner is paramount toward helping learners build on prior knowledge and skills. When beginning to consider integrating simulation into any curricula, it is often helpful to talk with faculty development professionals and other faculty who are familiar with the use of simulation in medical education. It is helpful to collaboratively explore opportunities for utilizing simulation; advantages of using simulation; and challenges to its implementation. An appropriate educational approach would be to consider what you want to teach, and then to consider the most appropriate way in which to teach it and whether simulation will assist the learner in achieving the learning objective. As is always the case in teaching, it is essential to establish goals and learning objectives, to determine the teaching strategies for meeting those objectives, and to determine whether the teaching and learning will be enhanced by the use of simulation; if and in what way simulation will support the teaching and learning; how simulation will be integrated into the teaching; and how its effectiveness (i.e., achievement of goals and objectives) will be evaluated. All are fundamental elements for teaching with simulation.

For example, consider whether it will help the learners move beyond memorization, help them to apply the new knowledge, and then transfer the information learned to real-life situations. As with the use of any technology, simulation is only a tool for teaching, it is not the curriculum. Gaba (2004) noted that the use of simulation can be categorized by 11 dimensions. Seven of these must be considered when designing and implementing any simulation experience, and are key to the effectiveness of the experience:

1. purpose of the simulation
2. unit of participation (e.g., individual, group, team)
3. level of the learner
4. healthcare discipline
5. type of simulation technology
6. degree of participation in the simulation
7. method of feedback.

Learning

As noted earlier in this chapter, simulation offers the learner opportunities to become engaged in experiential learning. Experiential learning "involves reflective thought, and influences subsequent actions and personal development" (Dunn, 2004, p. 18).

As described by Kolb (1984) (Fig. 7.1) experiential learning consists of four related components: concrete experience, reflective observation, abstract conceptualization, and active experimentation.

Figure 7.2 illustrates an adaptation of Kolb's (1984) model of experiential learning by Dunn (2004, p. 17), which identifies five points in the experiential learning cycle.

Dunn adds a fifth point to the cycle, that of "planning for implementation" – examination of what will be done differently in the next implementation. Thus, in Dunn's model, the learner moves from a concrete experience (an event), to reflection (what happened), to abstract (what was learned), to planning for implementation (what will be done differently), to active experimentation (what is done differently), and back to the concrete experience, thus completing the experiential and feedback loops.

Teaching and learning with simulation can use both the cognitive and psychomotor domains. Students move from acquisition of knowledge to demonstrating their ability to synthesize the information, and apply it to simulated and patient-based psychomotor experiences. Experiential learning operates with the principle that "experience imprints knowledge more readily than didactic or online presentations alone" (Dunn, 2004, p. 17).

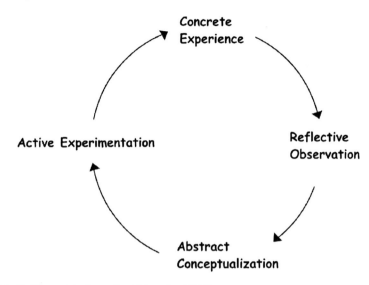

Fig. 7.1 Kolb's model of experiential learning (1984)

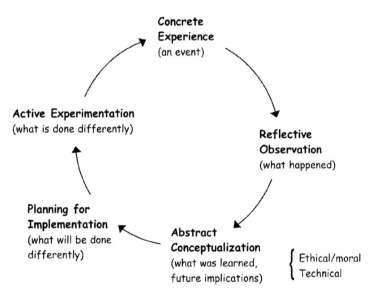

Fig. 7.2 Dunn's adapted model of experiential learning

Experiential learning offers the learner the opportunity to build knowledge and skills within the cognitive and psychomotor domains of learning. Bloom's (1956) hierarchy of learning in the cognitive domain has six levels of increasing difficulty or depth. Those six levels are:

1. knowledge
2. understanding (e.g., putting the knowledge into one's own words)
3. application (e.g., applying the knowledge)
4. analysis (e.g., calling upon relevant information)
5. synthesis (e.g., putting it all together to come up with a plan)
6. evaluation (e.g., comparing and evaluating plans).

Dave (1970) lists behaviors in the psychomotor domain, from the simplest to most complex:

1. imitation (e.g., patterning behavior after someone)
2. manipulation (e.g., performing actions with instructions)
3. precision (e.g., refining)
4. articulation (e.g., coordinating actions, achieving consistency)
5. naturalization (e.g., high level, natural performance)

Learning to apply previously acquired knowledge and skills to new contexts requires practice and feedback. Simulation provides teaching opportunities for integrating the basic and clinical sciences using problem solving and critical thinking, with the added benefit of facilitated reflection after the simulation experience, which, in simulation is referred to as debriefing. This will be addressed later in this chapter.

Building a Scenario

When building a scenario, it is important to keep the above detailed learning hierarchies in mind, and how they will be incorporated into the simulation scenario in order to optimally meet the needs of the learner. It will vary, depending on the stage of the learner. For example:

- Students learning facts and applying those facts to a new situation, such as might be the case in a foundational sciences curriculum in the early years of medical school.
- Residents learning a new procedure.
- Learners working on synthesizing information to develop a treatment plan, and evaluating that plan in light of other options.

In summary, one must be mindful of the level of the learner and the cognitive level the scenario is aimed at.

Simulation has the potential to bring life to teaching cases for learners at all levels of medical education. When developing a scenario, it is best to base the scenario on real cases and events, as they add robustness – as is true anytime one is teaching with cases. This is true whether developing a new scenario or adapting one for use in the simulation. It is important to design the scenario and develop teaching strategies

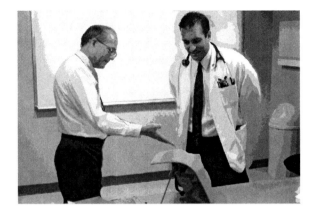

keeping the teaching goals and objectives at the forefront, so that confusing or non-pertinent content does not take away from the learning objectives. Additionally, it is important that every scenario have a clear take-home message, and includes an evaluation of learning.

Simulation technology can also be used in conjunction with standardized patients. Since many physical conditions cannot be replicated by standardized patients, simulation technology combined with the use of standardized patients is an approach for assessing learner performance and competence in some examination and other high-stakes testing situations. Integration of the two can also provide a more robust and realistic representation of clinical situations.

Components of an Effective Simulation Session

It is helpful to include four specific key components in every simulation session. Those components are: an introduction or briefing to the simulation session; the simulation itself; the debriefing; and an evaluation.

During the briefing, it is important that the faculty begin to create a climate of support and trust. It is also during this briefing component that the faculty share the purpose of the simulation, the basic elements involved, its goals and objectives, and what is involved in the debriefing process. It is also the time during which the ground rules for the simulation experience are set, as well as what is expected of the learners.

Key considerations for an effective simulation session include the following:

- select a limited number of educational points for each session
- take into account the level of learner and learning
- identify the resources needed
- prepare for the unexpected
- decide whether a co-facilitator for the debriefing is needed
- do a dry run prior to the actual simulation.

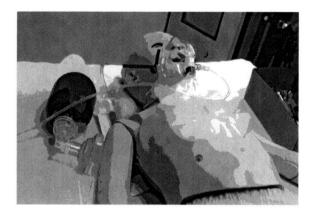

Debriefing and Fundamentals for Doing It Effectively

Debriefing is considered to be the essence of the simulation experience and is essential for the learning process. Debriefing occurs following the simulation and in a separate room from the simulation. The debriefing examines what happened (e.g., what was done well and what needs improvement), what was learned, and what will be done differently next time. It helps to identify and address gaps in knowledge; involves decisions about, and reflection on, the simulation, and often involves the viewing of a video recording of the simulation itself. Debriefing should be an interactive experience and beneficial to the learners, as well as the faculty.

When debriefing, it is important to keep in mind the goals and objectives of the simulation being debriefed; as well as the debriefing strategies. For example, will there be co-facilitators and what will their roles be? What will the strategy be for feedback and reflection? If video of the simulation was recorded, when and how will the video be used during the debriefing? The viewing of the video can be integrated into the debriefing in a few ways, but two frequently used methods are viewing the video prior to discussion and reflection, or viewing the video interspersed in the discussion and reflection for the purpose of emphasizing key learning points. Though review of video during the debriefing can allow learners to see what they actually did versus perception of what actually occurred, lengthy use of video can detract from the purpose and benefit of the debriefing component. The debriefing is facilitated by the faculty, but can also be co-facilitated by a learner whose role was observer of the simulation itself.

The established goals and learning objectives for the session are particularly key in helping the learner during the reflective aspect of debriefing. However, reflection on, and analysis of, an event is the foundation of experiential learning and within the process of experiential learning, debriefing is facilitated reflection. Reflective practice is a key factor in improving future practice.

To ensure an optimal debriefing experience for the learner(s), it is important that faculty conduct this component of the simulation keeping in mind the key elements of an effective debriefing, as well as those that detract from the debriefing process, as listed below (Dunn, 2004).

Elements of a successful debriefing:

1. create a friendly and confidential learning environment
2. provide pre-simulation expectations (e.g., simulator use and limitations, simulation principles, ground-rules)
3. encourage questions supportive of self-critique while fostering discussion
4. reinforce principles, correcting a limited number of errors
5. avoid excess correction, criticism
6. stress a key number of educational points
7. use visual aids, including the use of video, to review concepts or actions
8. avoid creating an excessively long debriefing.

Factors that detract from the debriefing process are as follows:

1. lack of an initial explanation of purpose, objective(s), orientation (e.g., of simulator)
2. excessive instruction discussion
3. closed questions and excessive criticism or negativism of learner's performance
4. consuming excessive time on medical issues
5. highlighting too many key teaching points
6. underestimation of trainee emotions
7. autocratic attitude of debriefer
8. allowing discussion to focus on the limitations of simulation.

The depth and length of debriefing needed in a simulation depends on factors such as the objectives of the simulation, the complexity, level of the learner, learner experience with simulation, time available, role of simulation in the curriculum, and relationship between the learners. It is particularly helpful when the debriefer critiques and challenges the learner while preserving a supportive, trusting relationship.

Faculty Development Considerations

Faculty development is an important component of any simulation program. Some basic skills needed include curriculum development (to include goals and objectives), teaching methods, scenario development, evaluation methods (including critical action checklists and other evaluation tools as needed), knowledge of simulation technologies, computer literacy, and debriefing.

Considering the importance of debriefing in teaching with simulation, as noted earlier in this chapter, it is critically important that faculty receive faculty development in debriefing methods and consider initially pairing with, or at least observing, an experienced facilitator.

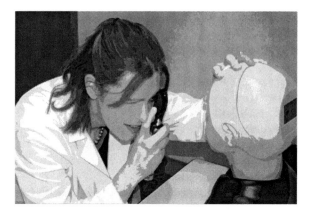

It is vital to the success of the simulation program to make faculty development and on-going support on teaching with simulation available to faculty via face-to-face and online programs. Such an approach provides an efficient and effective way to continually enhance faculty involvement in teaching with simulation and incorporate their feedback toward revising programming efforts. Moreover, it can potentially satisfy risk management continuing education requirements of health care professionals.

Faculty development is key toward helping faculty think about innovative and effective ways of teaching with simulation, and furthering the integration of simulation technology and effective learning. Moreover, it will advance the effective use of simulation as an existing and emerging instructional technology tool, and advance the assessment of technology-mediated student learning outcomes.

Summary

It is hoped that readers will be challenged to identify opportunities and potential applications of simulation in their curricula in ways that support teaching and learning; recognize benefits of using simulation; and begin to overcome any challenges to sound educational implementation. Teaching with simulation holds the ability to effectively help learners integrate the basic and clinical sciences, apply and integrate medical knowledge in a real-time and safe learning environment, practice without risk, and expand inter-professional communication and cooperation among healthcare professionals and throughout the medical school community.

References

Bloom BS, (Ed.) (1956) Taxonomy of educational objectives: The classification of educational goals. Handbook I: Cognitive domain. David McKay, New York.
Dave R (1970) Psychomotor levels. In: Armstrong RJ (ed) Developing and writing behavioral objectives. Educational Innovators Press, Tucson, AZ.

Dunn WF (Ed.) (2004) Simulators in critical care and beyond. Society of Critical Care Medicine, Des Plaines, IL.

Gaba DM (2004) The future vision of simulation in health care. Quality & Safety in Health Care 13(S1): i2–i10.

Gordon JA, Wilkerson WW, Shaffer DW, Armstrong EG (2001) "Practicing" medicine without risk: Students' and educators' responses to high-fidelity patient simulation. Academic Medicine 76(5): 469–472.

Huang GC, Gordon JA, Schwartzstein RM (2007) Millennium Conference 2005 on Medical Simulation: A summary report. Simulation in Healthcare 2(2): 88–95.

Kolb DA (1984) Experiential learning: Experience as the source of learning and development. Prentice Hall, Englewood Cliffs, NJ.

Ziv A, Wolpe PR, Small SD, Glick S (2003) Simulation-based medical education: An ethical imperative. Academic Medicine 78(8): 783–788.

For Further Reading

Dunn WF (Ed.) (2004) Simulators in critical care and beyond. Society of Critical Care Medicine, Des Plaines, IL.

This text is a robust and valuable collection of a spectrum of information and resources for those seeking to learn more about simulation in healthcare. Information ranges from program development to skills development and beyond.

Fanning RM, Gaba DM (2007) The role of debriefing in simulation-based learning. Simulation in Healthcare 2(2): 118.

This article offers the reader a review of literature on debriefing in simulator-based learning, as well as lessons learned from experienced facilitators. Though a useful resource for anyone involved in facilitating the debriefing process, it is particularly useful for those interested in enhancing their skills in this area.

Huang GC, Gordon JA, Schwartzstein RM (2007) Millennium Conference 2005 on Medical Simulation: A summary report. Simulation in Healthcare 2(2): 88–95.

This article provides readers with results of a 2005 inventory on virtual patient simulation activities at U.S. and Canadian medical schools.

Gordon JA, Oriol NE, Cooper JB (2004) Bringing good teaching cases "to life": A simulator-based medical education service. Academic Medicine 79(1): 23–27.

This article describes the development of an undergraduate medical education simulator program, including curriculum development and integration, and is an informative resource for readers seeking information in that regard.

Chapter 8
Teaching with Practicals and Labs

Travis P. Webb, Carole S. Vetter, and Karen J. Brasel

Over the last 50 years, medical education has seen an increase in time devoted to didactic teaching and a significant decline in the amount of time devoted to laboratory teaching and learning. The reasons for this are multifaceted, and the end result is not only unfortunate but ignores sound educational and learning theory. We hope that the fact that you are reading this chapter indicates your interest in reversing this trend and that you will find the information helpful as you incorporate laboratory exercises into your teaching repertoire.

Benefits of Laboratory Teaching

Laboratory teaching is one form of active learning, or the process of having students engage in an activity that forces them to reflect on ideas and how they are using those ideas. Knowledge is gained through a cycle of hands-on experience with reflection guided to conceptualization and then returning to application. When complemented by self-assessment the student's understanding and skill are further enhanced.

Laboratory teaching requires a change from teacher-focused lecturing to student-focused learning. Far from relieving the instructor from responsibility, laboratory teaching can increase the effort and time required of teachers, at least early in the transition from didactic lectures. The benefit? Increased student interest, attention, and knowledge retention. Most, although not all, studies suggest enhanced information transfer as evidenced by improved exam scores compared to students taught in didactic curricula. In addition, the majority of laboratory exercises are group learning events. This facilitates better solutions to problems, increased mastery of conceptual reasoning and retention compared to learning alone. These exercises can also develop critical skills in communication and team dynamics.

Laboratory teaching is often an opportunity to involve clinicians early in the science curriculum. The potential advantages are great – the students' education

T.P. Webb (✉)
Medical College of Wisconsin, Milwaukee, WI, USA

W.B. Jeffries, K.N. Huggett (eds.), *An Introduction to Medical Teaching*,
DOI 10.1007/978-90-481-3641-4_8, © Springer Science+Business Media B.V. 2010

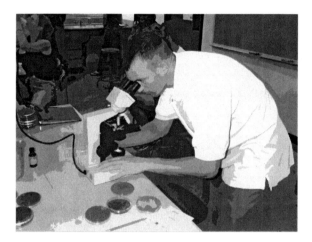

is enhanced by participating in an active learning exercise, the basic scientists are rewarded by interested and motivated students who can apply core concepts, and the clinicians benefit from early exposure to students, thus increasing student interest in their field.

Examples of Laboratory Teaching

Before we get into the nuts and bolts of how to conduct successful laboratory learning opportunities, here are a few examples of places they might be incorporated into an undergraduate medical curriculum. A word of caution – time in an undergraduate curriculum is scarce, and the addition of hours to an already overloaded schedule is often impossible. However, some schools have been able to use well designed laboratory teaching to decrease overall curriculum time. Creativity and cooperation among instructors along the basic science and clinical continuum are required to determine whether laboratory teaching is feasible, whether it can supplant current didactic curriculum, or whether it can be added without increasing student curricular hours.

Gross Anatomy

Clearly, gross anatomy is one of the prime examples of laboratory teaching, although it has changed with the advent of computer simulation and prosected models as many medical schools have moved away from cadaver-based dissection. This specific example pertains to a small exercise within the overall gross anatomy course. At our institution, clinicians, primarily surgeons, participate in the gross anatomy lab in order to focus the students on why learning anatomy is important. Several times during the semester, these clinicians come to the anatomy lab to demonstrate procedures on the cadavers – central line insertion, chest tube insertion, tracheostomy, and laparoscopic cholecystectomy. The students are given a handout before each session that describes both the technical details of the procedure and the relevant anatomy. Clinicians teach the procedure at the "bedside" of each cadaver, allowing interested students to perform the procedure. Clearly, the first year students will not become proficient in chest tube placement after this exercise. However, they have a better understanding of why time spent learning anatomy is important, and they sincerely appreciate the early interaction with clinicians.

Biochemistry/Physiology

A significant percentage of people with diabetes are unaware of their condition. The majority of medical students will treat patients with diabetes in their practice, and many will have the opportunity for initial diagnosis. To highlight some of the management issues facing patients with diabetes and teach about glucose metabolism, first-year students participate in a blood glucose lab in the biochemistry course in our curriculum. Students come to class after an overnight fast, learn how to use lancets to draw blood for measuring their own blood glucose, and take a baseline reading. They then eat breakfast provided for them, either high fiber, high simple sugar, or high fat. Glucose readings are taken throughout the morning, and students compare their glucose values with each other. Thus they are able to understand why dietary modification is an important part of diabetes management. They participate in discussions led by a diabetes educator, nutritionist, family practitioner, and biochemist.

A similar laboratory centered around the diagnosis and management of metabolic syndrome is held at the Indiana University School of Medicine. The initial lab teaches students how to draw blood from one another. Students then measure fasting blood triglycerides, high-density lipoproteins, glucose, blood pressure, and central obesity on each other. They are then randomized to eat a regular meal or a meal that follows the National Cholesterol Education Program Step I or II diets. Often with repeated measurements, discussion about physiological, nutritional, and behavioral components of the syndrome ensues.

Clinical Procedures Laboratory

There is a laboratory rotation at the Medical College of Wisconsin that was developed to provide students with sufficient exposure and experience in caring for patients with life-threatening disease. The rotation includes having the students read chest radiographs with examples of traumatic pathology, placement of chest tubes and performing a cricothyroidotomy in a mannequin, placing skeletal traction devices on one another, and reading computed tomographic scans. All skills are performed with a faculty instructor in a small group setting in the context of case-based scenarios.

The key to this type of lab experience is the integration of didactic discussion with the laboratory and simulation experience. Furthermore, allowing the students to work in small groups makes them active participants in the educational process. Providing students with multiple ways to learn the material increases their enthusiasm as well as their understanding of the concepts. Similar experiences exist in many other places; some may be an entire course or rotation, while others are smaller components of larger rotations that may combine several different learning experiences.

This is clearly not an exhaustive list. Other successful laboratory exercises include performing electrocardiograms during a cardiac physiology unit, measurement of pulmonary function before and after exercise to demonstrate respiratory physiology in action, participating in noninvasive ventilation to learn about various ventilator modes, and others. Orthopedic labs use power tools and clamps purchased at the hardware store, and porous hard foam to simulate bones.

Developing Goals and Objectives for Laboratory Teaching

It is tempting to jump on the laboratory exercises bandwagon based on enthusiastic student response and belief in a good idea. BEWARE – laboratory exercises are meant to be part of an educational program, and must have clear goals, objectives, and outcomes assessment. Without these, they might be fun, but may not result in improved knowledge or skill, and will certainly require precious faculty time. The following mnemonic is helpful in constructing objectives.

SMART Objectives (Features of Objectives)

1. Specific.
2. Measurable.
3. Achievable.
4. Realistic (or results oriented).
5. Timeframe.

Goals and objectives for laboratory teaching will depend on the level of the student and where the laboratory is placed in the curriculum. They will also depend on whether the laboratory exercise is designed to supplant or enhance current curriculum.

A couple of examples illustrate the range of possible objectives. In the case where the exercise is supplanting didactic, teacher-based learning, existing goals and objectives will likely need to be covered. In the case where the exercise is

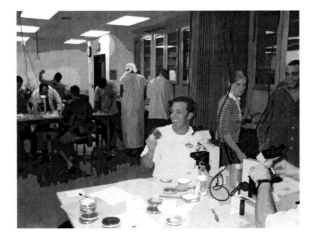

enhancing current curriculum, existing goals and objectives should be modified or additional ones developed. Several broad goals are possible, including skill acquisition, integration of basic science and clinical concepts, and early introduction of clinical faculty to medical students.

If the goal is skill acquisition, the objective would be demonstration of technical competence or proficiency. This is exemplified in the clinical procedures rotation above; the students are expected to demonstrate correct performance of a cricothyroidotomy and chest tube placement on a mannequin. For the clinician involvement in gross anatomy described above, the two goals do not relate to skill acquisition despite the fact that the laboratory experience is skill-centered. The goals of the lab are recognition of the importance of anatomy and early exposure of first-year medical students to practicing clinicians; the objectives are naming important anatomic structures relevant to each skill and individual conversations between students and clinicians. Similarly, the goal of the glucose lab is to understand the importance of diet and nutrition in the management of diabetes, with the objective of demonstrating differences in blood glucose after ingestion of different meals.

Assessment of Laboratory Teaching Exercises

It is important to consider assessment of student learning, or performance, as a well defined aspect of the educational experience. Both formative and summative assessment strategies may be applied to the laboratory setting. Assessment should be linked to the goals, objectives, and instructional methods in a manner that makes intuitive sense. If the objective is to identify the anatomic structures of the hand, then the assessment tool should include some form of labeling activity. For labs designed to teach skill acquisition, the appropriate method of assessment should be demonstration of the skill or a formal Objective Structured Assessment of Clinical Skill

Table 8.1 Matching of goals/objectives with assessment methods for lab exercises

Objective	Assessment method
Skill acquisition	Skill demonstration
	OSCE
	OSATS
Knowledge acquisition	Multiple choice examination
Decision making/critical thinking	OSCE
Influence or determine perception or opinion	Survey
	Questionnaire

(OSCE) or Objective Structured Assessment of Technical Skill (OSATS). If the laboratory exercise is designed to enhance knowledge acquisition, a traditional multiple choice question (MCQ) examination is sufficient. To assess deeper understanding and decision making, an OSCE can provide excellent formative and summative information. For laboratory exercises that are designed to influence perceptions, surveys or questionnaires are best (Table 8.1).

How to Set-Up a Lab Exercise

Laboratory set-up consists of two parts – instructor preparation and space/equipment considerations. Although space and equipment are clearly important, it is far more likely that instructor preparation will not get enough attention. Many teachers, comfortable with teacher-centered didactic instruction, will either not feel the need or not know how to do any preparatory work for a student-centered laboratory exercise. Inexperienced leaders of these exercises often make the assumption that facilitating student-centered learning is something that anyone who has been in an instructor/teaching role can do. The instructors or facilitators should receive a copy of the goals and objectives for the laboratory exercise, as well as the assessment tool, before the lab. They should be familiar with the conduct of the lab, and for a skills lab should be able to perform the skill with the available equipment. The students do not want to hear "well, this isn't really the way I do it" or "I'm really not sure why they are having you do it this way."

Instructors may need an instruction or refresher on "how to teach" active learning. A part of this introduction may need to address biases against active learning:

1. It lessens overall quality – the students could be listening to me lecture rather than doing this silly grade-school exercise.
2. Teaching does not occur unless knowledge is transferred from one individual to another.
3. An instructor's job requires that all material must be covered in the allotted time.

Specific behaviors that promote success in an active learning environment include:

1. Moving around the room and interacting with multiple students.
2. Asking directed or targeted, open-ended questions of specific students.
3. Asking students to reflect on what they have found, what it means, why it happens/happened.
4. Ensure that all students have a chance to participate.

Student preparation is also key. One of these tenets of active learning is that not all learning occurs within the classroom setting. The students should receive any necessary background material prior to the lab exercise, along with a copy of the goals and objectives of the exercise.

Space and equipment considerations and constraints may guide the lab design, although some may be lucky enough to be without constraints. Labs with a single user group require a larger space and less equipment; those with multiple smaller groups can make use of several smaller areas but require more equipment and most often more instructors or facilitators. Grounded electrical outlets with power from either ceiling or floor, special plumbing filters for biohazard material, sinks, freezers, work tables and cabinet space are all additional considerations. Demonstration videos are a nice alternative to live demonstration, particularly when expensive materials are needed; this requires specific AV and computer equipment.

Consumable supplies can be ordered, but can often be recycled from various places in the hospital. We work with our operating room and supply distribution center to appropriate all usable outdated or expired supplies. This helps keep lab costs down, always important but even more so if the lab is an addition to existing curriculum rather than a replacement. Other ways to reduce costs include collaboration between groups to use all parts of a cadaver and homemade simulators rather than commercially available ones. Wooden slats, plastic wrap, foam and foam tape make a reasonable "simulator" for teaching chest tube placement for a much lower cost than commercially available simulators. Additional options for lowering cost include sharing more expensive resources across several rotations.

Conducting the Lab

Now the fun begins! It is at this point that the focus switches from the teacher to the student and true student-centered, active learning occurs. Make the students commit to an answer prior to performing the exercise or lab – they will retain the information discovered during the lab much better when required to think through the problem and verbalize the answer beforehand. If possible, encourage the students to work in small groups to benefit from each other; however ensure that groups are not dominated by a single student.

For skills or procedures, an initial demonstration is imperative. Following the demonstration, some students will want to jump right in and others will want to observe a few more. To a point, this is fine, and likely reflects different learning

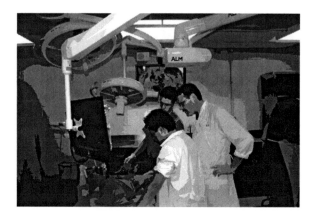

styles. The instructor's job is to ensure that each student gets enough opportunity to learn and practice. If a student is having difficulty, break the skill down into component tasks and demonstrate each one, having the student practice with immediate feedback.

A potential downside of a student-centered learning environment is that students will not discover or learn the particular point envisioned by the instructor. Under these circumstances you should re-evaluate the exercise and improve preparation. It's important to clearly delineate the objectives and assess how they will be met. However, problems may also be specific to a particular group of students, so don't change things too quickly. Gaps in achievement of lab objectives can be easily overcome by an attentive instructor. At the conclusion of the lab, the instructor should summarize to ensure that the key points have been made and all of the goals and objectives met. A short summation speech is one way to do this, although it can also be done by eliciting responses from the students and supplementing anything that is missed.

After the Lab

Similar to lab set-up, there are two aspects to consider after the lab is finished. First, the assessment must be complete – often an evaluation is worthwhile even if an MCQ exam or skills demonstration has been the primary method to assess the learner. Prepare good session evaluation forms to get feedback from both students and the instructor. This can be a tremendous help to improve future labs. Furthermore, these evaluations have importance in documenting academic scholarship for the instructors, thereby providing more incentive for faculty participation.

Supplies should be inventoried, and may need to be reordered prior to the next lab. Cleaning, maintenance, and ongoing evaluation of nonconsumable supplies are all necessary to determine whether capital expenditure is required for new equipment.

Pitfalls

The primary result of an unsuccessful laboratory exercise – whatever the reason for lack of success – is that the students will not learn what is intended. Almost all pitfalls are avoidable with a little preparation; it would be a shame to have the work invested in an active learning exercise not result in excited and accomplished learners (Table 8.2).

Table 8.2 Potential pitfalls in laboratory teaching

Pitfall	Undesirable outcome
Lack of goals and/or objectives	Waste of faculty time No learning occurs
Unprepared or uncomfortable instructors	Disinterested students No learning occurs Instructor attrition
Learning objective not covered	No learning occurs
No assessment strategy	Inability to judge success of experience Unclear if learning occurs

Summary

There are many opportunities to incorporate these exercises into medical education. With a little preparation, the change in focus from teacher-focused lecturing to student-centered active learning in a laboratory setting can benefit both.

For Further Reading

Fitzpatrick CM, Kolesari GL, Brasel KJ (2003) Surgical origins: New teaching modalities integrating clinical and basic science years-a role for residents as active teachers. Surgery 133(4): 353–355.

Glasgow SC, Tiemann D, Frisella MM, et al. (2006) Laparoscopy as an educational and recruiting tool. American Journal of Surgery 191: 542–544.

Graffam B (2007) Active learning in medical education: Strategies for beginning implementation. Medical Teacher 29: 38–42.

Gupta S, Westfall TC, Lechner AJ, Knuepfer MM (2005) Teaching principles of cardiovascular function in a medical student laboratory. Advances in Physiology Education 29: 118–127.

Kolb D (1984) Experiential learning: Experience as the source of learning and development. Prentice Hall, Englewood Cliffs, NJ.

Martin B, Watkins JB, Ramsey JW (2004) Evaluating metabolic syndrome in a medical physiology laboratory. Advances in Physiology Education 28: 195–198.

Martin BJ, Watkins JB, Ramsey JW (1998) Venipuncture in the medical physiology laboratory. Advances in Physiology Education 19: S62–S67.

Michael J (2006) Where's the evidence that active learning works? Advances in Physiology Education 30: 159–167.

Modell HI, Michael JA, Damson T, Horwitz B (2004) Enhancing active learning in the student laboratory. Advances in Physiology Education 28: 107–111.

Reiter SA, McGill C, Lawrence SL, Twining SS (2000) Blood glucose laboratory for first-year medical students: An interdisciplinary model for nutrition-focused diabetes management. Journal of the American Dietetic Association 100: 570–572.

University of Buffalo, National Center for Case Study, Teaching in Science, http://ublib.buffalo.edu/libraries/projects/cases (Cited 10/30/07).

University of Medicine & Dentistry of New Jersey, Center for Teaching Excellence, http://cte.umdnj.edu/active_learning (Cited 10/30/07).

Chapter 9
Teaching with Technological Tools

David A. Cook

The first use of educational technology probably occurred when someone picked up a stick and drew in the sand, or when someone picked up a piece of cinder and wrote on a cave wall. Chalk, papyrus, paintings, printed books, chalkboards, and more recently photographs, overhead projectors, televisions, and computers all represent technological advances that can used for educational purposes. It is common to become fascinated – or infatuated – with new technologies, but it is important to remember that these technologies are simply tools to support learning. No technology, no matter how sophisticated, will supplant a skilled teacher, effective instructional methods and designs, or – most importantly – the central role of the student in the learning process.

In recent years, computers have found an increasing role in medical education. Not only has computer-assisted learning (CAL) taken off, computers are now used to support face-to-face learning through the use of PowerPoint^{TM}, audience response systems, and multimedia (graphics, animation, sound and video). This chapter will emphasize such technologies, not because they are more important than or superior to older technologies, but simply because they are new and educators must become comfortable using them. However, teachers should consider all of the technologies available and use those methods that best serve the needs of the learner. The use of simulation is covered in another chapter in this book.

Fundamental Principles

Before discussing any specific technologies it is worth reviewing a few fundamental principles about how people learn, and also some principles about the effective design of multimedia presentations. These principles will be relevant to all of the educational technologies subsequently discussed, and are summarized in Tables 9.1 and 9.2.

D.A. Cook (✉)
Mayo Clinic College of Medicine, Rochester, MN, USA
e-mail: cook.david33@mayo.edu

W.B. Jeffries, K.N. Huggett (eds.), *An Introduction to Medical Teaching*,
DOI 10.1007/978-90-481-3641-4_9, © Springer Science+Business Media B.V. 2010

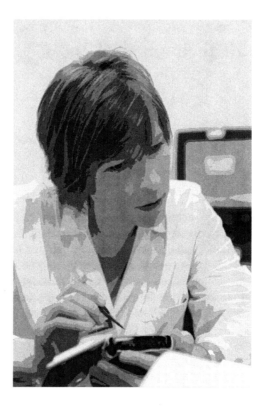

Core Principles of Instructional Design

As in all instruction, the use of educational technology should focus on helping learners effectively construct new knowledge rather than trying to effectively transmit information. Learning is more than accumulation of information, but rather involves organizing, reorganizing, and linking new information and experiences with prior knowledge and past experience. This process, known as elaboration, constitutes the core of all learning. Educational technologies will be most effective inasmuch as they encourage learners to construct robust, meaningful knowledge structures.

   In considering how to accomplish this, Merrill (2002) reviewed the literature looking for common themes among various educational theories and models, and distilled five "first principles of instructional design." First and foremost, all instruction should be situated in the context of real life *problems*. This is not synonymous with problem-based learning per se, but rather implies that patient cases (or other relevant problems) should figure centrally in all instruction. The second principle is *activation* – "learning is promoted when relevant previous experience is activated." Activation means that prior knowledge (including formal instruction and lived experiences) is brought to the forefront of working memory, where it can be integrated with new experiences and information. The third principle is *demonstration* – "learning is promoted when the instruction demonstrates what is to be learned, rather than merely telling information about what is to be learned." Next comes *application* – "learning is promoted when learners are required to use new knowledge or skills to solve problems." Guidance and coaching should be provided initially, and then gradually be withdrawn such that in the end learners can solve problems independently. Finally, *integration* – "learning is promoted when learners are encouraged to integrate (transfer) the new knowledge or skill into their everyday lives."

Designing Effective Multimedia

Based on decades of empiric research, Mayer (see Clark and Mayer, 2007) has formulated several principles of effective multimedia learning (Table 9.1). These principles are relevant to computer-assisted instruction, PowerPoint^{TM} presentations, and other uses of audio and video in instruction.

Multimedia Principle: People Learn More from Graphics and Words than from Words Alone

A picture is worth a thousand words, and it comes as no surprise that graphics, photographs, animations, and short video clips can greatly enhance learning. Graphics help learners construct effective mental representations. While irrelevant graphics actually detract from learning (see below), relevant graphics can be used to illustrate examples (and non-examples) of an object, to provide a topic overview or organization scheme, to demonstrate steps in a procedure or process, or to illuminate complex relationships among content, concepts, or time or space.

Modality Principle: When There Are Graphics, Present Words as Speech Rather than Onscreen Text

New information can reach working memory through separate visual and auditory pathways. Learning is maximized when both pathways are optimally used. For example, a graphic accompanied by spoken explanation (both pathways used) will be more effective than the same graphic accompanied by onscreen text (vision-only). Paradoxically, when identical information reaches working memory simultaneously via both vision and hearing (such as when a presenter reads their PowerPoint^{TM} slides verbatim) it can actually impair, rather then enhance, learning. Thus, the modality principle encourages teachers to maximize mental capacities by using both visual and phonetic information, while avoiding redundancy (presenting identical text onscreen and as speech).

Contiguity Principle: Related Information Should Be Placed Close Together

It is common to include an explanatory legend at the bottom of a figure. However, this physical separation of information wastes mental energy that could be better spent on learning. It is far more effective to place the explanatory text within the figure itself. This helps learners appreciate relationships (=build meaningful knowledge), and it minimizes the cognitive effort spent going back and forth between a figure and the accompanying text. The same principle applies to non-graphical elements, such as putting the directions for an exercise on the same page as the exercise itself, or presenting the question and the answer/feedback together when providing formative feedback on an online test.

Coherence Principle: Avoid the Extraneous (Less Is More)

Interesting but irrelevant details detract from learning. This includes sounds, graphics, or unnecessary words. Teachers often add cartoons or photos to presentations for aesthetic value (to "spice up" a lecture), but such decorative graphics can actually impede learning rather than enhance it. The same applies to extraneous sounds, interesting but irrelevant stories, unnecessarily detailed descriptions, and most animations. Not only does extraneous information tax cognitive capacities, it can also *distract* the learner from more relevant material, *disrupt* the learner from building appropriate mental links, and *seduce* learning by activating inappropriate prior knowledge which leads to flawed knowledge structures. The purpose of words, graphics, and multimedia in instruction is to help learners construct mental representations. If they do not serve this purpose, they should probably be removed. As John Dewey once stated, "When things have to be made interesting it is because interest itself is wanting. The thing, the object is no more interesting than it was before." (Dewey, 1913, p. 11–12) Bottom line: if it doesn't facilitate learning, leave it out.

Guided Discovery Principle, Worked Example Principle, and Expertise Reversal Effect

Many educators have advocated unstructured learning environments, claiming that freeing learners from the tethers of rigid instruction will enhance learning. However, abundant research suggests that this is not the case – at least, not all the time. The guided discovery principle states that learning is enhanced when information is presented in a planned sequence and when learners are assisted in their interpretation of this information – in short, when learners are guided in the learning process. This guidance need not be excessive. In fact, too much guidance diminishes the need for learners to think deeply about new information and weakens the resultant knowledge structures. The worked example principle is similar, namely that learning is enhanced when some practice problems are replaced with worked examples.

However, as learners advance they require progressively less guidance and become increasingly independent in solving problems. This transition from supported to independent learning and problem solving has been labeled the **expertise**

Table 9.1 Principles of effective multimedia learning

Principle	Learning is enhanced when ...
Multimedia principle	Both words and graphics (pictorial information) are used
Modality principle and redundancy principle	Descriptions of graphics are spoken rather than appearing as on-screen text, but concurrent written and spoken text are avoided
Contiguity principle	Related information (graphics and accompanying explanation; instructions; feedback) is placed close together (on the same page, and close together on page)
Coherence principle	Only necessary information (graphics, words, sound) is presented
Personalization principle	A conversational tone is used
Learner pacing principle	Learners can control the pace of the course
Guided discovery principle	Structure (content selection, sequencing, and interpretation) is present for novice learners
Worked example principle	Some (but not all) practice problems are replaced with worked examples
Expertise-reversal effect	Structure and worked examples are provided for novice learners, while advanced learners receive less structure and unsolved problems

See Clark and Mayer (2007) for details and additional principles of multimedia learning.

reversal effect. What works for novices will not work for more advanced learners, and what works for advanced learners won't work for novices. Learners should initially be provided guidance and worked examples, and progress to independence.

Educational Technologies as "Mindtools"

Jonassen (2000) has suggested that students should learn *with* computers rather than *from* computers. By this he means that instead of sitting in front of a computer tutorial, students should use computer-based tools such as word processing, spreadsheet, and database programs; programs to generate semantic maps; and online discussion as "Mindtools" to facilitate knowledge elaboration. Other educators have assigned learners to produce PowerPoint™ presentations, web pages, or video clips related to the topic of study. This paradigm – using computers and other technologies as knowledge organization tools, rather than tools for the transmission of knowledge – merits consideration and further research.

Faculty Training

A critical, but often overlooked, issue in the use of educational technologies is faculty training. Training needs include the technical and instructional skills (they are different!) required to develop an effective educational object such as a CAL

Table 9.2 General tips when using educational technologies

- Consider the need for educational technology: Are simpler technologies or traditional instructional methods adequate? Is this the *best* technology to meet the needs of this group/content/context?
- Spend less time/energy/money on bells and whistles, and more time planning for effective learner interaction
- Consider how you will stimulate active learning
  - Structure learning around a problem (e.g., patient case)
  - Activate prior knowledge, demonstrate, allow opportunity for application and integration
- Follow principles of effective multimedia learning
- Provide time for learning; set deadlines
- Practice or pilot the course before implementation

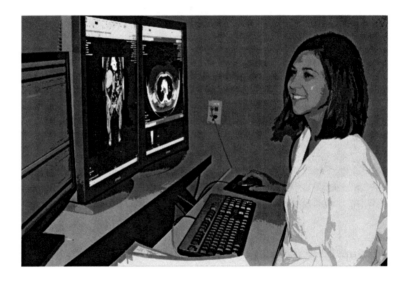

module, PowerPoint^{TM} presentation, or video clip, and the skills to integrate these objects effectively into a course. This chapter provides an introduction for faculty that focuses on the instructional aspects.

Computer-Assisted Learning

We will now discuss a number of specific educational technologies, beginning with CAL. CAL in all forms requires a paradigm shift for the teacher. Direct interaction with the learner is greatly reduced or eliminated altogether. However, the teacher continues to interact indirectly by virtue of the course/website design and the instructional methods selected.

There is nothing magical about CAL that makes it inherently better than other forms of instruction (such as face-to-face lectures or small groups). Decades of research have failed to detect any consistent advantage once changes in the instructional design/method are accounted for. Hence, educators should not jump to CAL as a solution for all instructional problems. Indeed, in many situations it is likely an inferior choice. Traditional methods or blended learning – using various combinations of CAL and traditional methods – are often the most effective approach. CAL comes in many flavors or configurations, including tutorials, online communities, virtual patients, performance support, online resources, and portfolios. Each of these will be discussed in turn.

Computer-Based Tutorials

What It Is

Computer-based tutorials are similar to face-to-face lectures. They consist of structured information, often enhanced by multimedia and interactivity. Such tutorials are often Web-based, although they can also be implemented on specific computers or using digital media.

When To Use

Computer-based (and in particular Web-based) tutorials have advantages such as flexibility in the physical location or timing of participation; the presentation of a consistent and easily updated message; learner self-pacing; facilitation of assessment and documentation; and a number of novel instructional methods that are difficult to implement in other modalities. However, there are also a number of disadvantages, including difficulty in adapting to individual needs; social isolation; development and maintenance costs; and technical problems. Computer-based tutorials will be most useful when learners are separated in time or space (such as conflicting schedules or rotations at different sites).

How To Use

When planning a CAL tutorial, it is important to do your homework. The initial development costs are likely to be great (perhaps much more than you anticipate), and this and other disadvantages should be balanced against potential advantages. Be sure that you have adequate technical support at your institution. Consider who will be doing the programming and who will provide technical support when problems arise. If commercial software meeting your needs is available, it may be cheaper to purchase this rather than develop a new program in-house. Proprietary learning management systems such as Blackboard or free, open-source systems such as Moodle can be helpful in organizing your course.

When developing the course itself, pay attention to the design principles noted above. In particular, remember that the goal of instruction is mental activity on the part of the learner – elaboration of information and construction of new knowledge. Physical activity (such as clicking the mouse) does not guarantee mental activity; direct your design to facilitate mental activity. Opportunities for self assessment and feedback, reflection, and interaction with other learners can facilitate this. Also, well designed interactive components can help. However, keep in mind the coherence principle – if it does not add to learning leave it out. Clark and Mayer (2007) provide additional considerations in thorough detail.

Also pay close attention to the website design. In addition to Mayer's principles, Web pages should be organized for consistency and clarity. Use the same basic layout from one page to the next within your course. Create a visual hierarchy to focus attention, and chunk related information together. Make it clear at all times, "What can I do on this screen, and where do I need to go next?"

Before implementation, pilot the website in terms of both functionality and appearance. Make the website readily accessible to learners. Secure commitment from all stakeholders – not just from the administration, but also from faculty and learners. Don't forget to provide time for learning. There is temptation to tack a Web-based course onto an already full schedule. CAL permits flexible scheduling, but does not prolong the hours of the day. Table 9.3 summarizes these recommendations.

Table 9.3 Tips for computer-based tutorials

- Use commercial software if it meets your needs
- Get buy-in from administration, faculty, and students
- Distinguish physical and mental activity: clicking mouse $\neq$ learning; try to stimulate mental activity
- Make site accessible and user-friendly

Online Communities: blogs, wikis, and discussion boards

What It Is

Internet-mediated communication has facilitated the development of so-called online learning communities. In the virtual equivalent of a face-to-face small group discussion, learners can interact to share experiences and information and learn collaboratively. As with face-to-face small groups, online learner interaction serves both a social function and as a stimulus to active learning.

Most online communication is asynchronous – there is typically a delay between sending a message and receiving the response. Tools for asynchronous communication include e-mail, threaded discussion boards, blogs, and wikis. Synchronous communication is real-time, and is mediated through Internet chat rooms and instant messaging. In a threaded discussion, a learner or facilitator makes an initial post on a specific topic to pose a task or a question for comment. Responses are grouped according to the message to which they are responding. One message might have five responses, and each of these responses could in turn have any number of responses. The discussion thus spread like paths diverging in a forest, yet the collective train of thought for any given path can be easily followed as one picks up one end of the "thread" and follows the conversation to the end. Blogs (short for web logs) consist of dated posts organized in reverse chronological order. There is no threading or branching, and often only one person (the author) contributes to the posts. Usually there is a provision for visitors to comment on the content of the blog. Wikis, from the Hawaiian word for quick, allow all users to contribute to revisions of the same document or web page.

When To Use

The advantages and disadvantages of online communities compared to face-to-face small groups are similar to those described above for tutorials. They will be most useful when learners are unable to meet together face-to-face (in fact, it is probably preferable for learners to meet in person when possible).

One might choose threaded discussion when the emphasis is organization of communication around specific themes or topics; blogs when the goal is documentation of personal impressions, such as e-portfolios (discussed in greater detail later on) or a journal; and wikis when the objective is a collaboratively developed final product.

How To Use

After deciding to develop an online learning community and selecting the appropriate configuration, the next step is to identify or train a qualified facilitator. Effective online small-group facilitation requires a unique skill set. The "e-moderator" must ask questions, challenge points of view, provide summaries and synthesis, redirect when a discussion goes astray, promote active participation from all group members, and encourage a healthy social environment. At the same time, the facilitator must remain a "guide on the side" and ensure that the learning evolves from group collaboration.

Online learning communities seem to work best when some degree of structure is provided. The facilitator will typically pose a question or specific task to the members of the group. For example, a problem-based learning task might give a group an unstructured case and ask members to analyze the case (see Chapter 4), identify problems, and come up with a solution. Case analysis is similar but emphasizes the identification of root causes of the problem rather than solutions, often considering multiple different paradigms or perspectives. Critical incident discussions ask students to identify a formative experience (such as an influential positive role model, or an error made in patient care) and identify salient details of this incident. Groups then identify common themes among their experiences.

It is often helpful to assign students to work in groups of two to five to ensure that everyone has an opportunity to participate. There are various permutations on this theme, such as breaking apart and reorganizing groups halfway through an assignment, encouraging participants to work as individuals initially and then collaborate for the final product, or begin as a group and then submit a final product written alone. Wikis allow groups to work collaboratively on a single final product. Firm deadlines should be fixed well in advance (on or before the first day of the course, if possible). Interim deadlines are useful as well.

It is often appropriate for the facilitator to post resources such as journal articles and book chapters (provided copyright law is taken into account), written introductions or summaries, slide presentations, or links to external websites. However, these should not supplant the collaborative group learning process.

Two serious threats to online communities are inflammatory communications between group members and silence. The first problem ("flaming") can lead to a loss of mutual trust and disintegration of the collaborative environment. Those involved in heated discussions should be redirected by the facilitator, and if this proves unsuccessful they may need to be excluded from participation. "Lurkers" read messages but do not post responses. Not only are such individuals less likely to learn deeply, but by failing to contribute they negatively affect the experience for all. After detecting lurking, facilitators should first try encouraging participation from all participants generally. If this is unsuccessful they may need to resort to one-on-one communication with the individual student.

Learners should be taught the rules of "netiquette" that govern online communication. First and foremost be polite. Learners should carefully proofread messages before posting and consider whether their words could be misinterpreted. Typos can be confusing, and small errors in spelling and punctuation can completely change the meaning of a sentence or paragraph. Writing in ALL CAPS is considered yelling and should be avoided. Empty messages such as "I agree" should be shunned in favor of more informative comments about *why* the individual agreed. Participants should carefully read what has been previously posted to avoid repeating comments. Humor should be employed with great caution: without voice inflection and physical gestures it is easy for messages to be misinterpreted. Finally, participate: all communication in the community should be done in a common forum (such as the discussion thread), except when personal feedback to an individual might be inappropriate for a group setting (such as from the facilitator to someone who is flaming or lurking). Table 9.4 summarizes tips for online communities.

Table 9.4 Tips for developing online learning communities

- Choose a configuration appropriate to learning goals: email, threaded discussion, blog, wiki
- Train the facilitator
- Assign tasks that promote meaningful collaboration and learning
- Develop the social aspects of the group
- Beware of lurkers and flaming
- Judiciously incorporate online resources such as websites, documents, multimedia, and slide presentations
- Teach "netiquette": participate, be polite (proofread messages, review for alternate interpretations, no personal attacks), avoid all capital letters, no empty messages

Virtual Patients

What It Is

A virtual patient is "a specific type of computer-based program that simulates real-life clinical scenarios; learners emulate the roles of health care providers to obtain a history, conduct a physical exam, and make diagnostic and therapeutic decisions" (AAMC Report, 2007). The defining feature (and limitation) is the attempt to mimic reality on a computer screen. Virtual patients can range from patient cases that develop linearly with occasional prompts for the learner to make decisions or request additional information, to complex simulations that branch in response to learner questions and actions.

When To Use

The evidence base regarding virtual patients is limited, and most recommendations are based either on extrapolation from other forms of CAL or on conjecture and expert opinion. The most appropriate role of virtual patients appears to be the development of clinical reasoning. Lectures and CAL tutorials are probably superior for the development of core knowledge, and standardized patients or real patients are superior for the development of history taking, examination, and counseling skills. However, a growing body of evidence suggests that there are no generic problem solving skills in medicine (or any other subject), but rather that problem solving skills (such as diagnostic reasoning or selection among management options – collectively termed clinical reasoning) involve a large amount of pattern recognition. Hence, the development of clinical reasoning requires a large number of patterns, which derives from seeing lots of patients. If real-life experience is insufficient, supplementing the mental case library with simulated experiences may help. Virtual patients provide an efficient way to provide such experiences.

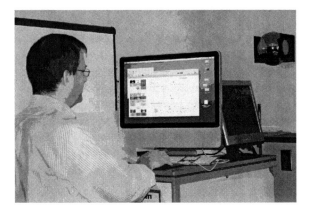

How To Use

The key consideration in teaching with virtual patients involves the selection, sequencing, and implementation of cases. Ideally, cases on a given topic would start off relatively simple (and perhaps with some guidance in decision-making) and progress to more challenging cases with greater complexity and less guidance. Looking to facilitate elaboration (which George Bordage [1994] has termed "the key to successful diagnostic thinking"), teachers might encourage learners to explicitly contrast two or more cases, to justify the elements of history, exam, and laboratory testing they select, to rank diagnoses in the order of probability, to explain how their choices might change with a slight variation in the clinical scenario, or to identify the evidence in favor of their management strategy. Feedback might consist of an expert's approach to the same case, an index of concordance with accepted guidelines, or measures of cost or time efficiency.

Regarding the design and implementation of virtual patients, technological sophistication does not equate with better learning. Much attention is paid to the fidelity or realism of the virtual patient. However, these concerns are likely ill-founded. Not only is high fidelity expensive, but there is some evidence to suggest that it can paradoxically impede rather than enhance learning. Likewise, while intuition suggests that asking learners to type questions into the computer to elicit a history may be most effective, evidence suggests that selecting questions from a preset list of standard questions may be more effective. Finally, many virtual patients require learners to click on specific body organs to examine them. It is unclear whether this activity enhances learning (mental activity) or merely represents physical interactivity.

The development of a good virtual patient library can be difficult. Not only are scenario scripts time-consuming to prepare, but the technology to turn a script into a working virtual patient can be expensive. Efforts such as the MedBiquitous virtual patient standards group and the AAMC's MedEdPortal are working to facilitate the sharing of such resources among institutions. Authoring tools such as CASUS and WebSP can help, and commercial products such as DxR Clinician should also be considered.

Even after cases have been developed, there is still the issue of how to integrate these into a curriculum. Some educators have found that working through a virtual case as a group is more effective than working alone, or that virtual patients are most effective as part of a blended learning activity (for example, having a face-to-face group discussion once everyone has completed the case). Additional considerations include: Will cases be mandatory or optional? What is the right balance between virtual patients and real patients? Are learners who have seen real patients with a similar problem able to opt out? How will learners find time to work on cases? What training will teachers need in the use of the software and specific cases, and how will institutional buy-in be achieved?

Just-In-Time Learning (Performance Support)

What It Is

Just-in-time learning involves delivering educational information at critical stages in a clinical encounter (performance support). Information can be "pushed" to the provider (such as automated feedback in response to specific triggers in computerized order entry, feedback linked with electronic prescribing patterns, or CAL packages that tailor their activity and response to individual practice patterns) or "pulled" by the provider (online searchable resources, personal digital assistants [PDAs], or smart systems that provide quick access to needed information). The essence is that the learner (who is often a practicing healthcare professional) can either seek, or be automatically provided with, information relevant to the patient sitting in front of them. The theoretical educational advantages are at least twofold. First, this is a moment when learners (practitioners) will be receptive to the material, since it (hopefully) will enable them to provide improved patient care. Second, because a knowledge gap has been identified and prior knowledge activated, learners are primed to integrate this new information into their existing knowledge structure.

When To Use

Just-in-time learning is used when learners (providers) are seeing patients. As useful as this sounds, it has limitations. It takes time to read, digest, and assimilate this information in a busy clinical schedule, and learners may resent mandatory pop-ups or unsolicited e-mail reminders if these affect their practice efficiency. Also, just-in-time learning may not substitute for other instructional approaches because the ad hoc, unstructured information may be improperly integrated. For example, a teaching point relevant to one patient may be over-generalized to a population for whom a different rule should apply; or the knowledge structure may be left with gaps not addressed by the performance support system. Thus, performance support – at least at present – is just that: support. It should not replace (at least not completely) other instructional methods.

How To Use

The paucity of evidence makes specific recommendations difficult; however the suggestions for CAL tutorials likely apply. Additional questions to consider include how much information to present, how to organize and structure this information to facilitate meaningful learning, how to motivate learning, and what will trigger the information to appear? Effective instructional methods (which usually take more time) must be balanced against the time constraints of a busy clinical practice. As evidence and experience accumulate performance support systems will likely become more prevalent in coming years.

Online resources such as Google™ and UpToDate have become the first line information source for many practitioners. However, the availability of such resources does not guarantee that they will be used, or used effectively. The same pedagogical concerns described for "pushed" information apply here. Furthermore, online resources raise the danger of unguided discovery – which, as noted above, can be detrimental for novice learners. The presence of misinformation on the Internet is another potential danger.

Portfolios and Online Assessment Tools

What It Is

An important part of teaching is learner assessment, and computers can facilitate this in numerous ways. The administration of online self-assessment and summative tests is now commonplace, and typically allow automated grading and immediate personalized feedback.

Education portfolios can include a variety of information and "artifacts" relevant to a student's professional development, similar to an artist's portfolio of completed works. Relevant information might include case reports, patient logs, records (written, audiotaped, or videotaped) of performance, essays, research project reports, and self-reflection narratives. Online tools can simplify such portfolios. Logbooks are a specific type of portfolio used to keep track of procedures performed and patients seen.

When To Use

Online self-assessments are useful as pretests, interim tests, or posttests to help learners identify strengths and knowledge gaps. Formative feedback can itself be a powerful instructional method. Online summative assessments can be used for grading and documentation in addition to providing feedback.

Portfolios are particularly helpful in assessing domains that do not lend themselves to multiple-choice tests, such as attitudes, critical thinking, application of theory to practice, and progress over time. Since students study what will be tested, portfolios provide one way for teachers to emphasize these important elements of training. Reflection itself is an important instructional method that can be facilitated by portfolios. Portfolios will likely see greater use as the limitations of existing assessment tools are increasingly recognized.

How To Use

Specific information on assessing student performance can be found in Chapter 11. Many commercial and open-source tools are available to facilitate online testing.

When considering an online portfolio, the first decision is what type of information you wish students to include. These materials should align with the objectives of the course or curriculum. Students will need clear guidelines about the type of materials to be included and the narrative or explanation to accompany each component. Deadlines are important. Clear grading criteria, aligned with the objectives of the course, will need to be established and shared with the student. Such criteria might assess the organization of materials; the amount of thought and reflection evidenced in discussion; and other criteria specific to the type of material included (such as scores on a multiple choice test, or scientific rigor in a report on a research activity). Faculty development may be needed for both the faculty members who assist the students in developing the portfolio, and also those who assign grades.

Software for the development of online portfolios could be as simple as a blog or a wiki, or the student's personal page in a learning management system, or a software package designed for this purpose. Personal digital assistants (PDAs) are now used for many portfolio purposes, including patient tracking and procedural logbooks.

PowerPoint

What It Is

For many decades, 35 mm slides were the primary presentation-support tool. Today, slides have been largely replaced by the use of PowerPoint^{TM}. In the 20 years since its first release this software has developed into a powerful and versatile presentation-support tool. Software (e.g., Camtasia^{TM} and Articulate^{TM}) is also available to turn PowerPoint^{TM} presentations into polished Web-based learning modules. Specially designed screens (Smartboard^{TM}) can seamlessly integrate whiteboard techniques (the traditional "chalk talk") with a PowerPoint^{TM} presentation.

When To Use

Although PowerPoint^{TM} presentations are ubiquitous today, they are often not necessary. In fact, for many teaching purposes an open discussion or use of a chalkboard or whiteboard may be more effective. PowerPoint^{TM} will be most useful for formal presentations, such as scientific reports, or when multimedia (particularly graphics and photographs) will enhance the teaching session. However, PowerPoint^{TM} is a tool – and as with all technological tools, can be overused.

How To Use

Developing a PowerPoint^{TM} presentation can be fun because of all the things you can do. However, first and foremost you should focus your time and energy on developing the content and organization of the presentation rather than the PowerPoint^{TM} slides. Think more about how to mentally engage the audience and less about how to execute PowerPoint^{TM} animations and transitions.

The principles described above for effective multimedia learning apply to PowerPoint^{TM} as much as they do to CAL. In particular, the coherence principle applies to the use of PowerPoint^{TM} slides. Most notably, slides should be simple. Use no more than five to seven words per line, and no more than five to seven lines per slide. This may not seem like a lot (and you've likely seen this principle violated frequently) but slides should list merely the key points. You, the teacher, will then elaborate on these points – but if you put full sentences or excessive information, the audience will begin to read your slides (a violation of the redundancy principle). If you must add a direct quote, put only a short excerpt on the slide.

Consistency is a virtue. Using the same fonts, font size, color scheme, and transitions, and even similar clip art styles, will enhance learning by minimizing distraction. The slide master (View → Master → Slide master) allows you to control default settings for the entire slide show. Never use a font smaller than 28-point. Avoid nonstandard fonts (fancy fonts are both harder to read and also may not be available on a different computer). Colors should contrast, but avoid garish combinations such as green on red. Dark text on light backgrounds is easiest to read. In addition, a light background lends itself to writing on the slide using a SmartBoard™. Each slide design (more below) comes with a palette of colors for text, title, accents, hyperlinks, etc.; try to stick with this palette rather than using other arbitrary colors. Finally, just because PowerPoint™ offers lots of options for fancy transitions and animations does not mean you need to use them. In fact, simpler slide shows – with "boring" standard transitions – are usually more effective. PowerPoint™ allows the use of multimedia including clipart, photographs, charts and diagrams, tables, sound, video, and hyperlinks to Internet sites. All of these are useful when used appropriately, but as with everything else can be overdone. Use them only when they truly enhance the presentation.

Presentations often take longer than you think; plan at least 1 min per slide, and time your presentation before presenting. Instead of reading slides verbatim, put only the key points on your slides and then elaborate on these as you talk. Face the audience (not your slides) when presenting. If you are using a video clip be sure to try it out on the computer system you will be using – you may find the clip does not run on a different computer or project well using a different projector.

Although detailed instructions on using PowerPoint™ are beyond the scope of this chapter, there are a few features that you may find useful. *Slide designs* allow you to choose from a variety of templates with background, colors, and fonts that have been selected (hopefully) because they work well together. As noted above, the *slide master* can help with consistency within the presentation. The *slide layout* feature has several standard text layouts, including a title slide, text slides, text and graphics, etc. *Custom animation* can be used to introduce certain elements of a slide in sequence (for example, if you don't want all of the text or graphics to be visible at once) but it should not be overused. Finally, the *speaker notes* (typing text below the slide that is not visible to the audience) can be invaluable both for organizing your thoughts, and also for when you come back to give the presentation again at a later date. Table 9.5 summarizes these and other tips.

Table 9.5 Tips for using PowerPoint

- Spend more time on the content and organization than on designing your slides
- Plan for interaction with the audience
- Follow the Coherence Principle:
  - o Just the essentials on slides (you'll fill in details verbally)
  - o Simplicity and consistency (use slide master and color scheme)
  - o Bullet points: 5–7 words per line, 7 lines per slide
  - o Large, simple fonts (no less than 28-point font)
  - o Colors: contrasting and vibrant but not garish
  - o Minimize transitions, animations, sound, and other effects
  - o Use clip art, pictures, sound, video, tables, and hyperlinks to support learning (not decoration)
- When presenting
  - o If using video: test in advance on presentation computer
  - o Practice and get feedback; time your presentation
  - o Don't read slides, and don't read *to* slides

Audience Response Systems

What It Is

Audience response systems (ARS) actively engage the audience in the lecture. Commercially available ARS provide each attendee a small keypad with which they respond to questions posed by the lecturer. Responses are relayed via infrared or radio frequencies to a computer that integrates responses and displays them immediately in a PowerPoint™ presentation. Another approach requires each attendee to have a laptop computer linked (typically via wireless) to a central network through which they can work collaboratively and interactively on a variety of projects. This latter approach requires greater infrastructure but also provides greater flexibility.

When To Use

ARS will be most useful when teaching a large audience; for smaller audiences verbal interactions might be more appropriate. An effective, interactive non-PowerPoint™ lecture probably need *not* be altered just to use a PowerPoint™-enabled ARS. Audiences may become complacent with ARS if they are overused.

How To Use

Complex questions will confuse the audience and derail the lecture. Thus, ARS questions should be short, simple, clearly written, and typically employ five or fewer response options. Questions should be used sparingly in the presentation – predominately to emphasize key points. Since the whole purpose is to encourage audience interaction, questions should be designed to stimulate discussion and time should be budgeted to permit such discussion. Transitions (introducing the question, presenting responses, initiating discussion, and then resuming the lecture) should be rehearsed. When lecturing in a new venue the ARS should be tested well in advance to ensure that everything works properly. If the audience is unfamiliar with the ARS, you will need to provide clear instruction on how to use the keypad. When teaching the same learners over time (e.g., a medical school course) consider assigning keypads and tracking individual responses. Table 9.6 summarizes these recommendations.

Table 9.6 Tips for using audience response systems

- Keep questions short and simple, and use ≤ 5 response options
- Use questions to emphasize key points and stimulate discussion
- Allow time for (and encourage) discussion of answers
- Rehearse, preferably in proposed location
- Provide clear instructions to audience
- Do not overuse

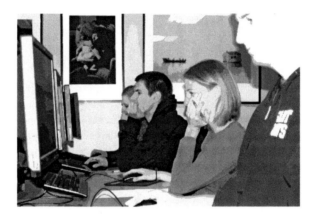

Similar principles will apply when using a more complex system (e.g., wireless network). Do not let fascination with the capabilities of technology take precedence over effective instructional design.

Video

What It Is

Video recordings for instructional purposes can range from brief clips integrated into lectures to full length feature films. Videoconferencing can allow a teacher at one location to reach an audience at another. Video archives or podcasts of lectures are increasingly commonplace. This section will deal primarily with the first of these uses, namely the use of video as an instructional technique.

When To Use

Video can be judiciously used to enhance any teaching activity. It can "reveal" the remote (separated by barriers of distance), the invisible (such as microscopic events or abstract concepts), and the inaccessible (unavailable due to risk or infeasibility). However, when experiences (such as lab experiments, patients, and procedures) are visible and accessible it makes sense to encounter them in person. Copyright issues should be considered before using video produced by others.

How To Use

First and foremost it is important to define the purpose for using the video. Video can be used to provide an overview or stimulate interest at the beginning of a course; to demonstrate principles, concepts, skills, procedures, or positive or negative role models; or as a "trigger" to self-assessment and critical reflection. Your purpose will define the type of clip, the length, and most importantly the way in which you use the material. A teacher may occasionally wish to show a full-length film, but more often short clips – preferably less than 5 min in length – will be more appropriate.

If learners are not encouraged to think before, during, and after the video the exercise will become a passive process (=ineffective learning). Careful planning will prevent this problem. Before starting the video, you should describe the context: the plot (especially if showing an excerpt from a longer film), the characters, and the setting. It is usually appropriate to provide an overview of what viewers will see and what they might learn, although in some instances this information might be withheld. It is always important to provide a specific objective and/or task to focus learners' attention. For example, you might suggest they watch for specific events; attend to dialogue, body language, or emotions; identify underlying assumptions, principles, or paradigms; or reflect on their own reactions and perspectives. Consider pausing the video midway to recap what has happened or ask learners to predict ensuing events, or try turning down the sound and narrating events. Discussion following the video should be encouraged.

Rather than using pre-existing video, learners might be video recorded during a role play with another student, an interaction with a standardized patient, or a procedure. This video can then be reviewed one-on-one or (cautiously, and with permission) as a group as a stimulus for self assessment, reflection, and formative feedback.

Recent developments in digital video have brought relatively sophisticated editing techniques within the purview of many educators. While a detailed discussion of specifics of videography is beyond the scope of this chapter, one useful online reference is provided at the end of this chapter. Table 9.7 summarizes these recommendations.

Table 9.7 Tips for using video

- Have a clear purpose – why are you using this clip?
  - o Reveal remote, invisible, or inaccessible
  - o Activate prior knowledge
  - o Demonstrate principle/concept/skill/procedure
  - o Trigger for discussion, self-assessment, reflection, attitude change
- Set the context (plot, characters, situation); consider providing an overview
- Focus attention: define objective (what can be learned) and/or task in advance
- Keep clips focused (typically <5 min)
- Encourage learners to think
- Pause to recap, discuss, predict next events
- Don't infringe copyright

Other Educational Technologies and Conclusions

This chapter could not begin to address all of the technologies available to educators today. Technologies such as overhead projectors, 35 mm slides, whiteboards and black boards, and printed materials are probably familiar to educators. Newer technologies include virtual microscopy, virtual cadaver dissection, and simulations of various kinds. Teachers are also using clinical technologies to enhance their teaching; for example, some medical schools perform whole body CT scans of cadavers prior to anatomy lab dissection.

Given these technologies and others not mentioned, educators are faced with an ever-growing toolbox from which to select specific instructional approaches. It is easy to become enamored with one or more technologies and forget the big picture. Educational technologies are only tools to help learners learn more effectively. Those who wield these tools should not only be skilled in their use, but must know when to use each one and when a different tool is needed.

References

Bordage G (1994) Elaborated knowledge: A key to successful diagnostic thinking. Acad Med 69: 883–885.

Clark RC, Mayer RE (2007) E-learning and the science of instruction, 2nd edn. Pfeiffer, San Francisco, CA.

Dewey J (1913) Interest and effort in education. Boston: Houghton Mifflin Co.

Jonassen DH (2000) Computers as mindtools for schools: Engaging critical thinking, 2nd edn. Merrill Prentice Hall, Upper Saddle River, NJ.

Merrill MD (2002) First principles of instruction. Educational Technology Research and Development 50(3): 43–59.

Summary Report of the 2006 AAMC Colloquium on Educational Technology (2007) Effective use of educational technology in medical education. Association of American Medical Colleges, Washington, DC, https://services.aamc.org/publications

For Further Reading

General principles

Clark RC, Mayer RE (2007) E-learning and the science of instruction, 2nd edn. Pfeiffer, San Francisco

Merrill MD (2002) First principles of instruction. Educational Technology Research and Development 50(3):43–59

Summary Report of the 2006 AAMC Colloquium on Educational Technology (2007) Effective use of educational technology in medical education. Association of American Medical Colleges, Washington, DC https://services.aamc.org/publications

Curriculum Repositories

Med EdPORTAL "http://www.aamc.org/mededportal" www.aamc.org/mededportal

Health Education Assets Library (HEAL) HYPERLINK "http://www.healcentral.org" www.healcentral.org

Merlot "http://www.merlot.org" www.merlot.org

Computer-assisted learning

Cook DA, Dupras DM (2004) A practical guide to developing effective web-based learning. J Gen
    Intern Med 19:698–707
Ellaway R, Masters K (2008) AMEE Guide 32: e-Learning in medical education Part 1: Learning,
    teaching and assessment. Med Teach 30:455–73; Part 2: Technology, management and design.
    Med Teach 30:474–89.
Ruiz JG, Cook DA, Levinson AJ. (2009) Computer animations in medical education: a critical
    literature review. Med Educ 43:838–46.

Online communities

Sandars J (2006) Twelve tips for effective online discussions in continuing medical education. Med
    Teach 28:591–3
Sandars J (2006) Twelve tips for using blogs and wikis in medical education. Med Teach 28:680–2

Virtual patients

Cook DA, Triola MM. Virtual patients: A critical literature review and proposed next steps. Med
    Educ 2009; 43:303–11.
Huwendiek S, Reichert F, Bosse HM, et al. (2009) Design principles for virtual patients: a focus
    group study among students. Med Educ 43:580–8.

Portfolios

Driessen E, van Tartwijk J, van der Vleuten C, Wass V (2007) Portfolios in medical education:
    why do they meet with mixed success? A systematic review. Med Educ 41:1224–33.

PowerPoint

Holzl J (1997) Twelve tips for effective powerpoint presentations for the technologically chal-
    lenged. Med Teach 19:175–9

Audience response systems

Robertson LJ (2000) Twelve tips for using computerised interactive audience response system.
    Med Teach 22:237–9

Video

Mitchell K Videography for educators. Available via http://edcommunity.apple.com/ali/story.php?
    itemID=365. Cited 9 October 2007

Chapter 10
Designing a Course

Christopher B. Reznich

"Dr. Samuels did that for years. Now that he's gone, we need a new EBM course. Can you take that on?"

Sooner or later, many of us who work in medical education will hear a variation of this quotation. A time will come when you'll be called upon to create a course. Unfortunately, many confuse a course with a list of topics or content to be covered. With the information in this chapter, you will be able to design a true course: a series of integrated instructional units that result in learner acquisition of knowledge, skills and attitudes.

There is a "trick" to designing a course. That trick is encapsulated in what Yelon (1996) has called "The Secret of Instructional Design." This is a depiction of The Secret (Fig. 10.1).

There are several principles represented by The Secret. All well-designed instruction contains certain elements:

- It meets an educational need.
- A description of the real world performance problem the course addresses, a course goal, an overall course objective, a visual model of the course units, and a description of the course content.
- Course units that lead learners to attainment of the course goal. Each unit contains its own objective, content, instructional/learning strategies, and learner evaluation strategies.

These elements must be consistent with each other. They must support each other and not clash or work against each other. This chapter will explain the elements of instructional design, and how they are integrated to be consistent with each other. But first, are you sure you have an "educational" problem?

C.B. Reznich (✉)
College of Human Medicine, Michigan State University, East Lansing, MI, USA

W.B. Jeffries, K.N. Huggett (eds.), *An Introduction to Medical Teaching*,
DOI 10.1007/978-90-481-3641-4_10, © Springer Science+Business Media B.V. 2010

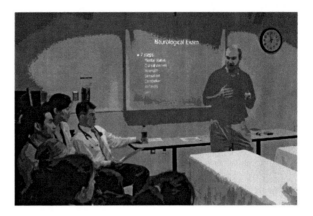

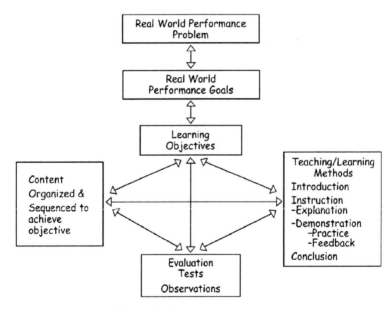

Fig. 10.1 The components of instructional design

First Steps: Needs Assessment and Feasibility

It takes a lot of time and effort to create a course. You want to be sure you need a course before beginning to work on one. Often, when there is a performance problem – your students or residents cannot do something competently – there is an automatic assumption that training or education is the solution. This isn't necessarily so! Consider the following scenario:

Dr. Mark has noticed that students in his program do not write post-encounter notes well. Important objective data are often missing, and assessment and plan sections do not follow logically from the data provided.

Dr. Mark decides that a brief course in post-encounter note writing is needed to make sure his students perform this task competently.

There are several possible reasons that Dr. Mark's students aren't writing notes appropriately:

- The students were never taught effectively, they simply don't know how to do it.
- The students know how to write notes, but they know that most preceptors will ignore their notes or give very cursory feedback.
- The students never have enough time to write notes well.

Which of these is a true "educational" deficit? If you answered "the first," go to the head of the class! Only those issues that are due to a lack of knowledge and/or skill are educational problems. Other factors might inhibit performance, including faculty system design or lack of motivation.

So, before setting out to develop a course or other form of instruction, make sure your potential learners really don't know something, or can't perform a task competently! How can you do this? Some good places to start include:

- Assess your learners on the desired knowledge and skills.
- Review any performance data you have.
- Review your curriculum for the presence or absence of the desired knowledge and skills.
- Review the literature to see if other institutions think this is a performance problem, too. This can also lead to some good educational ideas, if you decide to proceed with course design.

Even if you know you have an educational problem on your hands, you still need to think before you design:

- Do you have the resources you need to develop and implement your course? Most importantly, will you be given TIME, that most important resource, to devote to your course?
- Do you have the institutional support that will allow you to get the resources you will need to develop and implement your course?
- Do you have access to learners at appropriate times and places in your curriculum so that they can learn effectively and efficiently from your course?

The important question is: Is your course feasible? A well-designed course could fail because promised resources were not made available, or curricular time couldn't be spared to implement the course effectively. I know of at least one medical educator who spent 9 months developing a beautifully-designed, comprehensive course on medical informatics, only to see his professionally bound document gathering dust on the shelf when computers he was promised were not forthcoming!

How do you determine if your curriculum is feasible? Ask about critical resources (Bland et al., 2000):

- Ask the people in charge of scheduling at your institution if they are willing to give you time to develop and implement the course.
- Determine whether you will have access to your target learners in order to implement your curriculum.
- Figure out if you will have other resources such as space, equipment, staff, supplies and colleagues in order to implement your course.

Sometimes, even a good idea for a course, one that responds to a true educational need, must be put to the side because it isn't feasible. So:

- Be sure your performance problem is due to a lack of knowledge and/or skill, and
- Be sure your environment will support the development and implementation of your course.

The remainder of this chapter will explain the elements of The Secret of Instructional Design and their purposeful integration – how to make the elements consistent with each other.

Designing the "Big Picture" of Your Course

Designing a course is a lot like any design project. For example, in building a house, you need a plan, a set of blueprints that tell the builder where all the rooms go, the dimensions of each room, where the electrical fixtures, plumbing, windows and doors go. So much detail! But a good set of blueprints includes at least one that presents the picture, the overview that gives the builder and the buyer an idea of what the whole house will look like when it is finished.

When designing a course, you need a big picture, one that will allow your learners to know what the whole thing will look like and what to expect from the complete learning experience. This big picture serves several useful functions:

- It describes the real world performance problem the course addresses through a clear rationale for the course.
- It orients your learners to the course "destination" or goal, and the major course components and their sequence. This is often accomplished through a goal and a visible model of course units.
- It establishes course objectives, which inform your learners of how they will be assessed.

Let's look at each of these in turn.

Course Rationale

"Why do they have to learn this?"

Even if you have clearly defined a performance problem in your mind, that is no guarantee that your learners will see it as a problem! Smart course designers always cue their learners as to why a course was developed in the first place. This is often accomplished by including a rationale on the first page.

These are three elements of a course rationale: statement of the problem, cause of the problem, and exploration of why this course is the solution to the problem.

The combined statements, with support from the literature, form a complete rationale:

> "The ability to perform basic screening examinations is fundamental to physician training. Students at the Bien-Faire Medical College, have shown varying levels of competence at neurological and cardiovascular screening examinations due to differing levels of exposure to and practice with those tests.
> This course is intended to bring all entering interns to a standard level of skill in the neurological and cardiovascular screening examinations, irrespective of their backgrounds."

A brief paragraph or two modeled on the example will provide your target learners with the reasons why they should learn what your course has to offer them.

Course Goal

"What will they be able to do after they've finished this course?"

You've all heard the expression, "If you don't know where you're going, any road will get you there."

Pity the poor learners in courses that are just lists of topics! They often suffer from this problem, and have no idea what they are to do with all this marvelous content they've memorized.

As discussed in Chapter 1, a well-designed course provides learners with a clear destination in the form of a **course goal**: the knowledge and skills as they are applied in the real world to solve the problem presented in the course rationale.

In order to develop a course goal, ask yourself the following question:

What will your learners know and be able to do in the real world after completing your course?

Your answer to this question should contain the following elements:

a. A role for your learner ("As a third-year student. . .")
b. A context for applying the knowledge and skill (". . .as a clerk in the ambulatory clinic. . .")
c. A statement of learner behavior or performance upon completing the course (". . .the student will be able to perform a neurological screening examination when called upon.").

Again, putting the pieces together, you have the following examples of course goals:

"A third-year student, as a clerk in the ambulatory clinic, will be able to perform a neurological screening examination when called upon."

An easy way to remember the purpose of a goal statement is to recall that:

"G" = "G"
"Goal" = "course Graduate"

A goal specifies what a "graduate" of the course should be able to do in real life when the course is completed.

You might be confused by the reference to "real life" behavior or performance here. "Real life" will vary considerably, depending upon your referent system: your learners and what you intend for them to do when they finish your course. "Real life" for a pre-clinical medical student may be the ability to take vital signs and communicate effectively with patients during their clerkship years, after they've completed their first two years of training. Real life for a resident may indeed refer to their independent practice of medicine after they have completed your course and all of their residency training.

Remember to specify what your learners should know and be able to do, and in what context, after they have finished your course.

Course Objectives

"What are the measurable learning outcomes required to achieve the course goal?"

The course goal describes what your learner will know and be able to do when they have finished your course. But, how will YOU know that your learners have learned, and will be ready to perform in the real world? You will know by assessing your learners in some manner. Student assessment should be as close an approximation to real life as possible, to ensure that your learners will be able to perform appropriately in the real world. A complete array of assessment possibilities is discussed in Chapter 11.

Example

For this goal: "Students who complete the course will be able to interpret the results of a urinalysis," consider these two assessments:
Assessment A: On the final exam, students are given a 25-item multiple choice test covering urinalysis test results.
Assessment B: On the final exam, students are given a series of urinalysis test results, and are asked to interpret them in writing.

Of the learners who do well on either Assessment A OR Assessment B, which would you trust to interpret urinalysis test results correctly in the real world? Those students who performed well on Assessment B, and thus showed evidence of the desired goal behavior, could reasonably be expected to perform this mental skill. For those students who did well on Assessment A, well, we'll just have to wait until we see how they interpret such test results in the real world first! On the other hand, students will probably have to do well on Assessment A before they do well on Assessment B, so Assessment A could be an "enabler" for Assessment B.

In the big picture of your course, it is important to inform your learners of how they will be assessed. This creates a set of expectations for your learners, and helps them to know what is needed to succeed in your course. We all want our learners to succeed!

Objectives should inform learners about the content of the assessment. This can include:

A description of the assessment (what will be given to learners, and what learners will be able to use). This can refer to test forms ("Students will be given a 50-item multiple choice test of concepts related to the pathophysiology of pain") or various assessment stimuli ("Students will examine three simulated patients").

A description of the desired behavior (what learners will be expected to do during the assessment). The important concept here is that learners' behavior should be either observable ("students will perform a complete history and physical examination"), or recorded ("students will record their answers on the forms provided").

A description of the criteria (what will be used as the ultimate authority for assessments). This can be expressed as a source ("according to the information found in Robbins, et al." or "according to the content presented in the lectures and the course pack").

A description of your lower limit, or passing score (how well learners will need to perform in order to pass). This can be expressed in terms of quality, or how well a learner performs ("at least 90% answered correctly" "with all checklist items performed" "so well that no pain is reported" "so well that no scar is left") or time, or how long it takes to complete the test ("learners will be given 50 minutes for the test" "the encounter must be completed within 20 minutes").

Here is an example of a complete course objective:

"Students will be given 5 copies of real urinalysis test results with patient information blacked out. Students will write an interpretation of each set of results, according to the handouts and lectures provided during the course. To pass, students will have to provide complete and accurate interpretations of all normal and abnormal test results. Students will have 60 minutes to complete the test."

What would happen if you left out:

The test situation? ("5 copies of real urinalysis test results") – students might not practice with real test results, or might not practice urinalysis test interpretation at all.

The test behavior? ("interpret in writing") – students might not practice written urinalysis test interpretation.

The test criteria? ("handouts and lectures") – students might use different sources to prepare for the test, which could lead to insufficient practice.

The test lower limits? ("complete and accurate interpretations, 60 minutes") – students might not practice as hard as they should.

By including well-developed course objectives, you tell your learners exactly what you expect them to do in order to perform well in assessments, thus creating the conditions that will maximize their chances for success.

Visual Model

"What does this course look like?"

All courses divide into parts. These parts are often called units, modules, or lessons. By dividing your course into parts, you will structure all the knowledge and skills your learners need to learn into meaningful, digestible pieces.

A visible model will allow you to show how your course is organized, how the parts relate to each other and to the whole course. Take a look at the following example (Fig. 10.2):

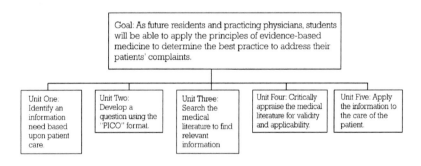

Fig. 10.2 Chronological order model

The course goal appears in the upper-most box. Note the role, the context, and the learner behavior specified in the goal. Each of the five units beneath the goal contributes something directly toward attainment of the goal, and each unit includes both a verb (behavior) and an object. This allows you to specify clearly your expectations of the learner.

In this case, the units are arranged chronologically, in the order in which they would be performed as a complete skill. There are other ways in which you can order your units in your visible model, for example (Fig. 10.3).

This model presents a framework for a clinical encounter, which will then be applied to a six different presenting patient symptoms. The basic skill set

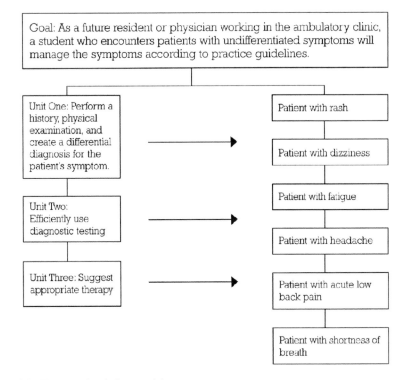

Fig. 10.3 Theme and variations model

remains the same: performing a history and physical examination (Unit One), efficiently using diagnostic testing (Unit Two), and suggesting appropriate therapy (Unit Three). This is the theme applied to six variations found in the differing symptom presentations. It is not important that students see patients in the order shown by the boxes of symptoms on the right-hand side; what is more important is the order of the tasks on the left-hand side.

Chronological order and "theme and variation," are two possible ways of depicting your course in a visual model. What is most important is to develop a display of your curriculum units that (1) accounts for everything your learners will learn in a systematic manner, and (2) shows how the various pieces of your course fit together.

Content Outline

"What are the knowledge, skills and attitudes that learners need to know?"

"Content" refers to the knowledge and skills you want your learners to acquire. As you design the big picture of your course, develop a brief content outline for each of your units. Do this by determining what is essential in order to learn the knowledge and skill described by the course goals and objectives.

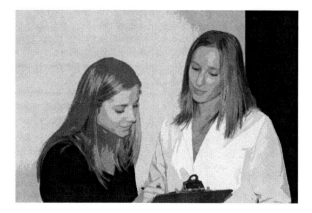

Example

Goal: As future residents and practicing physicians, students will be able to apply the principles of evidence-based medicine to determine the best practice to address their patients' complaints (Table 10.1).

Note that all the content specified in the column to the right is critical to attainment of the behaviors in the column to the left. There is nothing like "history of medical informatics" or other irrelevant content.

Let these principles guide you as you choose content for your course (Table 10.2).

Table 10.1 Sample content outline

Units	Content
Unit One: Identify an information need based upon patient care.	Identifying an information need: • Sources of information needs • Simple formats • Keeping a log of questions • "Hunting" and "foraging"
Unit Two: Develop a question using the "PICO" format.	Defining the patient (P) Defining the intervention (I) Defining the control or comparison (C) Defining the outcome (O)
Unit Three: Search the medical literature to find relevant information	Searching bibliographic databases (Medline) Searching web portals (e.g., WebMD) Searching compendia (e.g., Cochrane) Appropriate use of search engines (e.g., "Google Scholar" versus "Google")
Unit Four: Critically appraise the medical literature for validity and applicability.	Appraising articles on diagnosis, prognosis, and therapy
Unit Five: Apply the information to the care of the patient.	Models of patient education Health literacy

Table 10.2 Guiding principles for selecting course content

"Principle of shame"	Include only the **essential** knowledge and skills your learners need to **know** when they have completed your course – you would be ashamed if they didn't know this, or couldn't do this!
"Nice to know"	Content that may be related, but if left out it will not hurt learner attainment of the course goal. If you really want to include "nice to know" content in your course, do so as "supplemental reading" or appendices.

Your content should be as "lean" as possible. The predominant tendency among experts is to "teach" more, with learners feeling overwhelmed, as if they are "drinking from a fire hose." If you really want your learners to learn, less is often more! Less content will leave more time for meaningful practice and application of that content – but more on that when you begin to design your units.

Moving from the "Big Picture" to Designing Individual Units

Your "big picture" contains the elements described in Table 10.3:

Table 10.3 Elements of course content

Element	Function
Course Rationale	Describes the topic your course addresses, why that is an educational issue and how your course is the solution to the problem. Helps to motivate your learners.
Course Goal	Describes what learners who have completed your course will know and be able to do in the real world. Helps to orient and motivate your learners.
Course Objectives	Helps to establish course expectations. Informs assessment criteria.
Visual Model	Shows the different "pieces" (lessons, units, modules) of your course, how they are related, and how they lead to attainment of the course goal. Also helps to orient your learners.
Content Outline	Lists the different knowledge and skills that your learners will need to acquire in order to attain the course goal. This helps to establish course expectations for your learners.

Once you have a well-developed course big picture, you can begin to design the specific pieces of your course – the units, modules, or lessons. I use these words interchangeably, so we will use "units" for the remainder of the chapter. The next section will present a brief overview of how to design course units that will help your learners to acquire the knowledge and skill they need to attain the course goal.

Designing Your Course Units

As described earlier, each unit contains its own goal, objectives, content, instructional/learning strategies, and learner evaluation strategies. The remainder of this chapter will guide you through the steps in designing the unit components. Much of what you have already learned when designing the big picture of your course can be applied to designing your units. If you follow the guidance provided in this section, you will be able to develop a plan for your units that will guide you in creating the presentation and evaluation materials for that unit.

Unit Goals

As you did when designing the big picture of your course, you need to describe what your learners will be able to do in the real world after they finish a unit of instruction. The same elements you created when writing your course goal also apply to writing a unit goal: a role for the learner, a context for applying the knowledge and skill learned, and a statement of real world behavior or performance.

You will probably recognize this goal from one of our visual models presented earlier:

> Goal: As a future resident or physician working in the ambulatory clinic, a student who encounters symptomatic patients will manage the symptoms according to practice guidelines.

The visual model also specified three instructional units: (1) perform a history, physical examination, and create a differential diagnosis for the patient's symptom, (2) efficiently interpret diagnostic testing, and (3) describe appropriate therapy. The knowledge and skills in these units are applied to patients with different types of symptoms, e.g., patients with rash, patients with dizziness, etc. Since the unit titles specify a behavior, we can easily create unit-level goals from the unit titles:

> Unit 1: As future residents or practicing physicians, when presented with a symptomatic patient, the student will perform a history, physical examination, and create a differential diagnosis for the patient's symptoms.
> Unit 2: As future residents or practicing physicians, when presented with a symptomatic patient, the student will efficiently interpret diagnostic testing.
> Unit 3: As future residents or practicing physicians, when presented with a symptomatic patient, the student will suggest appropriate therapy.

Depending upon your own design sense, you may word your goals differently. For example, unit goal 1 may be split into three separate goals, one addressing history-taking, one addressing physical examination, and one addressing differential diagnosis. Like their big picture siblings, each unit goal includes a role, a context, and a description of the real world behavior or performance.

Unit Learner Evaluation

Evaluation of learners is addressed elsewhere in this book. Nevertheless, it is useful to introduce a guiding principle that will help you when you are designing your course instructional units.

If you know your unit goal, it is relatively easy to determine how best to evaluate your learners. The ultimate test of learning is performance of the knowledge and skill in the real world, under real world conditions. To the greatest extent possible, your assessments of learners should be realistic. For example:

If your goal is:

Students will be able to suture a wound leaving no scar.

Then your "best test" should be:

The student sutures a wound leaving no scar.

This represents an ideal learner evaluation; learners who pass this test will have our confidence that they can do the skill in the real world.

While this may sound logical, it is not always feasible to assess learners in the real world, under real world conditions. Therefore, we often try our best to create a close simulation of the behavior described in the goal:

The student must suture a pig's foot, employing the proper technique that will assure leaving no scar.

While we may not be as confident of a student who passes this test being able to perform the suturing skill in the real world, we are reasonably confident that she can ... but we'll be sure to observe her first real life performance!

Remember the principle: assess your learners under real world conditions, or under conditions that closely approximate the real world.

Unit Objectives

After you decide how you will evaluate your learners, you can write your unit objectives. Recall that an objective is a measurable learning outcome that is required to achieve the course goal. Thus it specifies the assessment situation, the assessment behavior, the assessment standards, and the assessment criteria.

Here is the objective from our "symptoms" course that accompanies the Unit 1 goal:

When provided with a written case scenario (test situation):

a. Students will state the history, signs and symptoms associated with serious causes of back pain, physical exam and psychosocial screening needed in a patient with acute low back pain (assessment behaviors).
b. Students will write a differential based on age, history and physical exam findings (additional assessment behaviors).

   c. They will then choose tests used in the evaluation of acute low back pain and explain
     their reasoning (additional assessment behaviors).
   d. Finally, the student will create a treatment plan addressing patient education, medication
     and non-medication therapy, activity limitation, exercise, case management and when to
     refer (additional test behaviors) using current practice guidelines (standards).

Any student reading the objective should have a good idea what the unit assessment will look like. From this example, it should be apparent that objectives can be of considerable length, as long as they serve the purpose of describing the assessment.

One can write objectives that describe assessments of a wide variety of knowledge and skill. For example, objectives can be used to describe assessments of interpersonal skill:

   Given 5 simulated patients, the student will obtain histories using the SPIKES protocol.

Objectives can be used to describe assessments of knowledge:

   Students will be assessed with a 90-item multiple choice test of pathophysiology, pharmacology, and microbiology related to the neuro-musculoskeletel system. Passing level will be set at 75% of items correctly answered.

Objectives can even be used to describe assessments of attitudes:

   Students will conduct interviews with 3 simulated patients, using the techniques specified in the course manual, and demonstrating respect for the patients according to the principles outlined in the manual. The interviews will be rated according to the checklist in the manual, with all mandatory items present in each.

Unit objectives follow the same guidelines as do course objectives. They are comprised of the same components, and serve the same purpose: to describe the assessment so that learners will have clear expectations as to how they will be evaluated.

Unit Content

What will be taught in each unit? The unit objectives specify the knowledge, skills and attitudes needed to accomplish the unit goals. But what will the unit actually teach? This is the unit content. Here are some content types, their definitions, and examples to consider, based loosely on the work of Robert Gagne (1985), a well-known learning theorist (Table 10.4).

Gagne's is an example of one way of analyzing the content of instruction, and there are others. Many in medical education are familiar with "Miller's Pyramid," which addresses clinical performance (Miller, 1990) (Fig. 10.4).

While Miller's evaluation framework was developed with assessment of clinical performance in mind, it is a useful framework for any complex skill set.

- *Does (Action)*: Individual functioning independently in practice.
- *Shows How (Performance)*: Can document what learner /trainee will do in real world setting.

Table 10.4 Types of knowledge and skills

Type of content		Definition	Examples
Knowledge	Facts	Organized collections of propositions	Different types of radiology imaging technologies and their strengths and limitations
	Concepts	Definitions/exemplars and examples	Diagnosis of different neurological diseases: examples include multiple sclerosis, hematomas, hemorrhages, dementias, and their defining characteristics
	Principles	Variables and their relationships: supporting evidence	
Skills	Psychomotor	Coordinated muscle skills	Taking a blood pressure Suturing
	Interpersonal	Communication and social interaction skills	Taking a culturally-sensitive medical history
	Intellectual	Using symbols to perform a task	Calculating a therapeutic dose

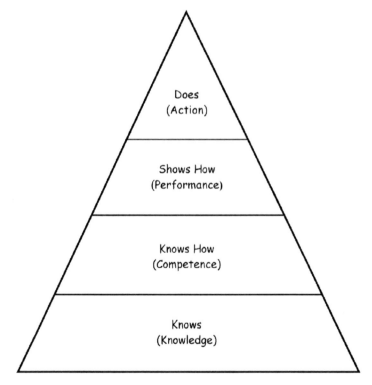

Fig. 10.4 Miller's pyramid

- *Knows How (Competence)*: Appropriate application of knowledge, skill in acquiring information, analysis, interpretation, creation of plans. Done in an academic setting.
- *Knows (Knowledge)*: Evaluation of knowledge base.

There are a variety of ways of conceiving content. As you think about your course, try to specify clearly what are the knowledge and skills you expect your learners to learn. It is important to have a sound idea of the different kinds of content you want your learners to acquire because, as we will see in the next section, that will make a difference in how they are taught and learned.

Unit Instructional Methods

A better word for this section would be "Unit Learner Practice Methods." The ultimate purpose of any unit instructional method should be to promote learner practice of the unit content. Too often, we conceive of teaching as "presenting" – lectures, grand rounds, noon conferences. Whatever presentation methods we use should not be ends unto themselves, but means to help learners practice.

Here is a simple way to conceive of instructional methods that includes student practice, with an example (Yelon, 2001):

- *Explaining the content*: present a video of how to do cardiopulmonary resuscitation (CPR).
- *Demonstrating how the content is used*: use a mannequin to show students up close how to deliver CPR.
- *Allowing time for learner practice of the content*: adjourn to a practice room where students take turns giving CPR to mannequins.
- *Providing feedback on learner performance of the content*: instructor observes student performance giving CPR, and provides corrective feedback.

As mentioned before, instructional methods may vary, depending upon what is being taught (Table 10.5).

While one may quibble with certain tasks or their details (e.g., "We have people who do our screening for us!") certain principles should stand out:

- All instructional methods should specify the means by which students should practice using the content.
- Practice should mirror how learners will be assessed.

By applying these two principles governing your choice of instructional methods, your learners will be guided to practice the content meaningfully, and should be well prepared to accomplish the objectives.

Table 10.5 Examples of instructional methods

If you want students to learn how to:	Then you should:
Recall the imaging capabilities of different imaging technologies, including their strengths and weaknesses.	Present an organized description of the capabilities of different imaging technologies, and their strengths and weaknesses. Demonstrate how you would memorize and recall the organized description. Present a table or mnemonic device that would promote memorization of these facts. Have your students practice recall in class, by quizzing each other after a few minutes of study. Test your students on their recall of the capabilities of different imaging technologies, and their strengths and weaknesses.
Perform cardiologic screening tests effectively.	Have students read description of the procedure for correctly performing the screening test. Demonstrate the cardiologic screening test procedure. Instruct students to pair up and practice the screening procedure on each other, with a third student observing and providing feedback. Assess your students on their ability to perform the test.

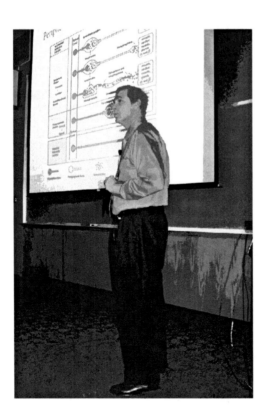

Final Notes

By following the guidelines in this chapter, you should be able to design a good plan for your course, one that is complete with respect to instructional elements, and in which the instructional elements "make sense" – they are tightly integrated with each other and aligned with the goal of the course. There will still be a lot of work to do! Lectures and other presentations must be developed, tests and test directions will have to be created, resources such as readings, presentation slides, labs, and simulated patients will have to be procured or developed as needed. Keep your plan in mind as you proceed with the development of your course.

It is advisable to get your course plan reviewed by experts in both the course content and in instructional design. Some questions you might ask of both types of experts are found in Table 10.6:

Table 10.6 Questions during expert review of your course

Questions for a content expert	Questions for an instructional design expert
Is the content I've specified for my course essential and up-to-date?	Is my design consistent?
Have I left out anything important?	Are my assessments a reasonable approximation of the tasks/behavior in my course goal?
Have I included anything that is not important and could be deleted?	Does the content appear appropriate for my objectives and assessments?
	Are my instructional methods appropriate for my objectives and assessments? Have I clearly specified how my students are to practice the content?
	Are there ways in which the design of the course could be improved?

By taking a systematic approach to designing your course, one that accounts for all instructional elements and their consistency with each other, you will be able to develop a course that is truly responsive to the educational needs of your learners.

Acknowledgements This chapter was based upon the work of the Primary Care Faculty Development Fellowship Program, College of Human Medicine/Michigan State University, William Anderson, PhD, Fellowship Director (HRSA Grant #D55HP00055).

I would also like to acknowledge Stephen L. Yelon, PhD, Professor Emeritus, College of Education, and fellowship faculty, Michigan State University, for use of his conceptual framework and for reviewing an early chapter draft; and Darryl Patterson, MD, former fellow, for the use of his course example.

References

Bland CJ, Starnaman S, Wersal L, Moorhead-Rosenberg L, Zonia S, Henry R (2000) Curricular change in medical schools: How to succeed. Academic Medicine 75: 575–594.
Gagne RM (1985) The conditions of learning and theory of instruction. Holt, Rinehart and Winston, New York.

Miller GE (1990) The assessment of clinical skills/competence/performance. Academic Medicine 65: S63–S67.
Yelon S (2001) Performance-centered instruction: A practical guide to instructional planning for trainers. Michigan State University, East Lansing, MI.
Yelon S (1996) Powerful principles of instruction. Longman, New York.

For Further Reading

Kern DE, Thomas PA, Howard DM, Bass EB (1998) Curriculum development for medical education: A six-step approach. Johns Hopkins University Press, Baltimore, MD.

Chapter 11
Assessing Student Performance

Brian Mavis

Assessment bridges the gap between teaching and learning. Perhaps second only to teaching, assessing student performance is a fundamental role in the life of a teacher. Assessment is important because it provides students with feedback about their performance; this information reinforces their areas of strength and highlights areas of weakness. Using this feedback, students can direct their study strategies and seek additional resources to improve their performance.

From the perspective of the teacher, another equally important function of student assessment is providing evidence necessary for decisions about student progress. The various student assessments within a class define the types and levels of achievement expected of students. As part of a course of study, student assessments describe a developmental process of increasing competency across a range of domains deemed necessary for graduation.

Any thoughtful teacher realizes the important role that student assessments play in their lives as teachers as well as in the lives of their students. Less obvious are the principles of educational measurement underlying sound student assessment practices. The purpose of this chapter is to provide an overview of some of the key features to consider when choosing among various student assessment strategies. This chapter will also provide information on how to create fair student assessments, that is, assessments that are both reliable and valid.

Reasons for Assessing Student Performance

As stated above, the assessment of student performance provides feedback to students about what they have or have not learned, and provides information that teachers can use in student progress decisions. However, these are only two of many possible goals that can influence your selection of student assessment strategies. As you can see by the list below, the goals that can drive the selection of student performance measures are many and far reaching:

B. Mavis (✉)
College of Human Medicine, Michigan State University, East Lansing, MI, USA

W.B. Jeffries, K.N. Huggett (eds.), *An Introduction to Medical Teaching*,
DOI 10.1007/978-90-481-3641-4_11, © Springer Science+Business Media B.V. 2010

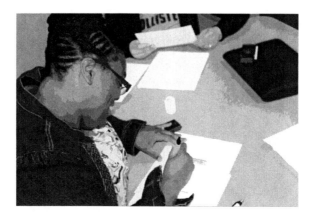

- Providing feedback to students about their mastery of course content
- Grading or ranking students for progress and promotion decisions
- Offering encouragement and support to students (or teachers)
- Measuring changes in knowledge, skills or attitudes over time
- Diagnosing weaknesses in student performance
- Establishing performance expectations for students
- Identifying areas for improving instruction
- Documenting instructional outcomes for faculty promotion
- Evaluating the extent that educational objectives are realized
- Encouraging the development of new curriculum
- Demonstrating quality standards for the public, institution or profession
- Articulating the values and priorities of the educational institution
- Informing the allocation of educational resources

Clearly, many of these goals are related directly to the interaction between teacher and student. Nonetheless, this same information can be used by other stakeholders in the educational process for a variety of other important decisions. From a practical perspective, it is unlikely that any single assessment strategy can provide information to support more than a few of these goals. The likelihood for misinterpretation or inaccuracy increases when student assessment data are used for purposes other than those originally intended. The sheer breadth of the list of goals above also demonstrates the importance of considering the use of multiple strategies to assess student learning.

In the curriculum development cycle presented in Chapter 10, student assessment follows instruction and is the impetus for reflection, evaluation and curricular improvement. While this cycle might reflect how many teachers approach teaching, from the student perspective, it is the assessment phase of the curriculum that drives learning. This is most often manifest when students ask, "do we have to know this for the test?" For many students their motivation is survival, and in an educational setting, one key element of survival is passing the test, whatever form student assessments might take. This is particularly true when results from assessments will be used for student progress decisions.

Learning the Language of Assessment: A Few Definitions

Before getting much deeper into a discussion of student assessment, it is important that we clarify a few definitions of key terms and their meaning in this context.

Assessment Versus Evaluation

Both assessment and evaluation refer to processes of gathering information for the purposes of decision-making. In medical education, assessment most often refers to the measurement of individual student performance, while evaluation refers to the measurement of outcomes for courses, educational programs or institutions. Practically speaking, students are assessed while educational programs are evaluated. However, it is often the case that aggregated student assessments serve as an important information source when evaluating educational programs.

Formative Versus Summative Assessment

Formative assessments are used to give students feedback about their learning. Practice test questions or problem sets, in-class peer-graded assignments and reviews of video recorded simulated patient encounters are examples of frequently used formative assessment strategies. Formative assessments are most valuable when they are separated from summative assessments, so that they are perceived to be low threat performance experiences. For conscientious students, this represents an opportunity to document both strengths and weaknesses. However, some students might dismiss formative assessments for their lack of consequences, and not put their best effort forward to use these experiences to maximal advantage.

Summative assessments are used to gather information to judge student achievement and to make student progress decisions. These assessments are very familiar to students and teachers, and for students often provoke anxiety. A substantial component of this anxiety comes from the student progress decisions that are predicated on performance. However, to the extent that uncertainty about the summative assessment strategy itself is a source of anxiety, teachers can take steps to reduce student anxiety. This includes providing information about the types of assessments to be used, their timing within a course, how they are scored and how each contributes to the final grade or progress decision. Students often become anxious in an unfamiliar assessment situation, such as a standardized patient encounter or new computer-based testing software. Sample interactions, in-class demonstrations or opportunities for non-graded practice can help students anticipate what to expect under these circumstances, which might help reduce their anxiety.

Competence

It is increasingly common in medical education for discussions of student assessment to lead to discussions of competence. One current definition of competence provided by Epstein and Hundert (2002) gives us a sense of the tip of the iceberg implied by these discussions. They wrote that "professional competence is the habitual and judicious use of communication, knowledge, technical skills, clinical reasoning, emotions, values and reflection in daily practice for the benefit of the individual and community being served." From the practical perspective of an educator, competence requires us to set expectations of satisfactory performance appropriate for the students' progress within the curriculum.

This approach to thinking about competence has been articulated by George Miller (1990), who has described a developmental model that is helpful when thinking about appropriate forms of learner assessment. For novice learners, competence is determined by what students *know*, i.e., their mastery of factual knowledge. At the next level, competence is defined by an assessment requiring students to demonstrate what they *know how* to do, such as how to use and apply knowledge to solve new problems, or demonstrate the clinical skills necessary to gather clinical data. At the next level, *showing how* in an assessment setting would be required to demonstrate competence. Assessments at this stage would require students to actually demonstrate their ability to acquire, interpret and translate knowledge. At the highest levels of competence, students would demonstrate competence by *doing*, which would be assessments of how they perform in an encounter with a patient in a real world setting.

Key Features of Student Assessment Methods

There are a number of factors to consider when choosing a method of student assessment. Attention to these factors at the planning stage will go a long way to helping you create a high quality student assessment. Five factors to consider are:

1. *Reliability*
2. *Validity*
3. *Feasibility*
4. *Acceptability*
5. *Educational Impact.*

Reliability and validity are characteristics that generally refer to the development of an assessment. Feasibility, acceptability and educational impact more often reflect contextual features of the assessment, which are related to when and how an assessment method is implemented.

Reliability

When talking about the reliability of an assessment method, we are referring to the consistency or repeatability of measurement. In practice a reliable assessment should yield the same result when given to the same student at two different times or by two different examiners. One of the advantages of tests comprised of multiple-choice questions is that they are highly reliable: the results of the test are unlikely to be influenced by when the test is administered, when the test is scored or by who does the scoring. Hence the term "objective" is often used when referring to these kinds of assessments. On the other hand, reliability is an important concern when grading essay questions, rating clinical skills or scoring other assessments requiring judgment or interpretation. In these situations, clear scoring criteria are needed to attain a high level of reliability, regardless of whether one or multiple people will be involved in grading the responses. Writing clear test questions and test instructions are important strategies for improving the reliability of an assessment by reducing the likelihood that test questions are ambiguous to the reader and open to multiple interpretations. Writing clear test questions also increases the likelihood that the assessment is testing desired knowledge, skills or attitudes rather than reading proficiency or verbal reasoning skills.

Internal consistency is another form of reliability that is more often used to describe assessments based on multiple-choice questions. This term refers to the coherence of the test items, or the extent to which the test questions are interrelated. The primary difference between this and other estimates of reliability is that calculations of internal consistency involve only one administration of the test. For example, a set of multiple choice questions focused on assessing students' knowledge of childhood immunizations should have high internal consistency. When questions testing other knowledge or abilities are added, the internal consistency is lowered. Internal consistency estimates are frequently provided as part of the output for machine-scored multiple choice tests. The concept of internal consistency can be applied to other methods of assessment; this is best done in consultation with a measurement specialist.

Validity

Validity is the extent to which an assessment measures what it is intended to measure. Validity is related to reliability, insofar as a test that has low reliability will have limited validity. A test with low reliability is subject to biases in interpretation and scoring, and when these biases are unrelated to specific content or student performance, the validity of the assessment is diminished.

Among the many types of validity discussed in education and social science research, content validity is the approach most commonly used to assure quality in student assessment. Essentially, an assessment is valid when it samples representatively from the course content. A common method for assuring that the assessment content is representative of the course content is to develop a table of specifications, often referred to as a test blueprint. The blueprint organizes course content by course objectives, such as students' ability to recall factual information, understand concepts or apply knowledge to new problems. Another approach to organizing content could be based on patient cases (well child visit, asthma, developmental delay, etc.), or by disciplines (pathology, physiology, pharmacology, nutrition, etc.). In reality, any organizing structure that reflects the logic of the course content can be used as the basis of the blueprint (Table 11.1).

Table 11.1 Sample blueprint for a clinical competence examination

Clinical competency	Case 1	Case 2	Case 3	Case 4	Case 5	Case 6
Communication skills	x	x	x	x		x
History-taking		x	x	x		x
Physical examination		x	x	x		x
Data interpretation			x	x	x	
Assessment/diagnosis			x	x	x	x
Patient education	x					
Written record	x		x	x	x	x

Ideally, the course content was initially designed around a blueprint based on the course objectives. In this way, the organization of the course informs the organization of the assessment content, creating a valid assessment. In situations where there are no preexisting course objectives, it might be necessary to derive them from the content and reverse engineer a blueprint prior to creating the assessment.

Content based on a blueprint approach works well for assessments that focus on recall and application of knowledge. This approach also can be extended to assessments of clinical skills. The specific steps used to teach communication, history-taking and physical exam skills define the content, and a rating form can be developed to judge student performance of these skills. Another approach frequently used for the assessment of skills is expert judgment. A number of practitioners or "experts" can be polled to determine what they would identify as the key components of a specific skill, and this consensus is the basis for the checklist developed to rate student performance.

In general, sampling assessment content from the same blueprint that was used to define instructional content can enhance the validity of an assessment. It might be necessary to use multiple methods of assessment when complex performance is the focus of assessment. Further, some assessment methods are more appropriate for some types of performance than others, so choosing appropriate methods can increase validity.

Feasibility

The feasibility of an assessment method is a judgment of the resources needed to implement it in light of the information to be gained. The development of a multiple choice test requires significant time in the development phase for question writing, but requires relatively little effort for administration or scoring. Conversely, a comprehensive assessment of clinical skills might require as many resources for scoring as for development and implementation, though the types of resources required might be different for each phase. Essentially, any assessment requires time for development, implementation and scoring. Additional resources might include examiners and/or simulated patients, as well as training time for each. Proctors, computers, biological samples, clinical case information, curricular time and building space are among other possible resources that can facilitate or constrain an assessment.

Acceptability

Consider a teacher weighing the use of three assessment strategies: weekly tests, a more traditional mid-course and final exam, or a single cumulative examination at the end. Each approach has its merits as well as limitations, depending on the purpose of the assessment. The acceptability of an assessment is based on the responsiveness of faculty and students to the assessment. If the assessment requires too much time from faculty and staff or requires too many resources to implement, the long-term survival of the assessment is jeopardized. Similarly, an assessment approach might be aversive to students because of the timing, length, content or other features. When this occurs and students do not prepare as expected for the assessment or do not see it as valuable to their education, the validity of the assessment can be jeopardized.

Educational Impact

The impact of an assessment is the sum of many influences. The intent of the assessment relative to the course objectives is a consideration. The thoughtful use of both formative and summative assessments can positively affect student learning and subsequent student performance. Educational impact also reflects the appropriateness of the match between the content and the assessment method; a mismatch reduces the educational impact. Since content and assessment method are linked, the use of multiple assessment methods can enhance the impact. Relying on a single method tends to focus assessment on the content most amenable to the method. The method can also influence how students prepare for an assessment, such as the differences in preparation for a multiple choice exam versus a standardized patient encounter.

Choosing an Assessment Method

Consider this example. As part of the neuroscience curriculum, second-year medical students were asked to identify the location of a lesion based on a written case included as part of their final examination, constructed from multiple-choice questions. The correct response was chosen by 88% of the class. The next day when the same question was presented in a different format within the context of a simulated patient encounter only 35% of the class got the answer correct. The conclusions about student performance based on each assessment would be very different. This example reflects the impact of assessment method in terms of both format and cognitive demands on the student.

When choosing an assessment method, there are several factors to consider. One of the first considerations is the type of performance to be assessed: is the assessment focusing on knowledge, skills or attitudes? Another factor that might influence the choice of assessment method is whether it is being used for formative or summative assessment. A related concern is the reliability and validity of the method. Some methods are more practical than others when considering the resources required to achieve reliable and valid results. Another consideration is whether more than one assessment approach should be used. When choosing an assessment method, it is important to remember that no single method "does it all." For this reason, a multiple-methods approach will probably provide a more accurate picture of student performance or achievement than relying on a single approach. As educators this idea makes intuitive sense; in practice we tend to stick to what is familiar.

The chart below summarizes the relative strengths of various assessment methods when measuring different types of performance. The chart provides guidance in choosing assessment methods, but is not intended to be absolute in matching methods and performance (Table 11.2).

Methods of Student Assessment

There are a wide range of methods available when developing your approach to student assessment. Presented below are assessment methods most common to medical education and while not exhaustive, this list represents a wide range of options available to faculty. The methods described in this section are organized into four broad categories: assessments based on written exercises, assessments derived from faculty ratings of performance, simulation-based assessments, and methods of global performance assessment. Each of the methods is described in terms of (a) strengths, (b) limitations, (c) reliability and validity and (d) construction tips.

Written Exercises

- Multiple choice questions (MCQs)
- Extended matching questions
- Short answer questions
- Essays and structured essay questions

Faculty/Preceptor Assessments

- Faculty global ratings
- Faculty checklist ratings
- Oral examinations

Table 11.2 Strengths of various assessment methods

Types of student performance

Assessment methods	Knowledge recall	Knowledge application	Communication skills	History-taking skills	Physical examination skills	Procedural skills	Professionalism	Team work	Written documentation	Attitudes	Self-reflection
Written exercises											
Multiple choice questions	X	X									
Extended match questions	X	X									
Short answer questions	X	X									
Essay questions		X							X	X	X
Faculty/preceptor assessments											
Faculty global ratings			X	X	X	X	X	X	X		
Faculty checklist ratings			X	X	X	X	X	X	X		
Oral exams	X	X							X	X	X
Simulated clinical encounters											
OSCE/standardized patients			X	X	X	X	X	X	X	X	
Technology-based simulations					X	X		X			
Other global assessments											
Peer assessment		X	X				X	X		X	
Self-assessment			X				X	X		X	X
Portfolios		X	X						X	X	X

Simulated Clinical Encounters

- Standardized patients and OSCEs
- Technology-based simulations

Other Global Assessments

- Peer assessments
- Self-assessments
- Portfolios

Multiple Choice Questions (MCQ)

Assessments based on multiple choice questions (MCQ) are one of the most common approaches to measuring student performance. Typically, a multiple choice question consists of two parts: the question (stem) and the possible answers (response options). Most MCQs include four or five response options and the student is asked to choose the best response. The stem also can make reference to tables, graphs or other information sources that the student must use in order to determine the correct response.

Which of the following best describes the path of air into the lungs of humans?

- (a) Alveoli, trachea, bronchi, bronchioles
- (b) Trachea, bronchi, bronchioles, alveoli
- (c) Bronchi, bronchioles, trachea, alveoli
- (d) Trachea, bronchioles, bronchi, alveoli
- (e) Alveoli, bronchioles, bronchi, trachea

Strengths

- Multiple-choice questions are familiar to most students, given their common usage throughout most levels of education.
- MCQs provide broad coverage of content. It is relatively easy to build an examination using MCQs that covers a wide range of course content.
- MCQs can be simply written to test for recall of factual knowledge, or can make reference to graphs, tables or illustrations to test cognitive skills. MCQs also can be posed within the context of a science problem or clinical case to test knowledge application and problem solving.
- Scoring of MCQs is highly reliable and objective.
- Scoring of MCQs can be automated, making scoring efficient and reducing the turnaround time for feedback to students. Automated scoring also facilitates the calculation of psychometric properties of each MCQ.

- MCQs are more flexible than True and False questions, which require absolute statements. MCQs are more flexible in terms of absolutes since the student is asked to choose the best answer from several possible options.

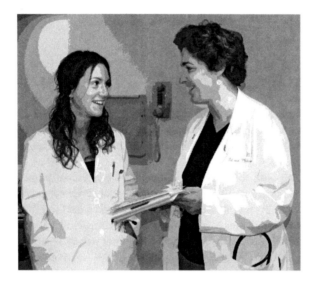

Limitations

- Good MCQs are challenging to write, especially for applications beyond knowledge recall such as knowledge application and problem solving. The time saved in scoring a MCQ examination is usually required up front in the preparation of the questions, which requires time to construct to avoid cueing students about the correct response option.
- MCQs frequently focus on recall of factual information and rely on students' recognition of the correct answer from among the options provided.
- Guessing can be a successful test-taking strategy for those questions where the student can rule out a number of the response options.
- MCQs are limited as a means of providing instructive feedback to students since usually the only information provided is the correct response option.
- The ease of use and economy of scoring associated with MCQs can lead to their overuse in situations when other types of assessment would be more appropriate.

Reliability and Validity

- Reliability tends not to be an issue for MCQs, which are the most frequently used objective test format. MCQ scoring is highly reliable in terms of consistency from one time to the next as might occur if the exams are scored over several sessions.

Scoring is consistent between examiners; scoring of MCQs is not dependent on who is scoring the exams.
- Validity of an exam based on MCQs is enhanced through the use of a test blueprint, which assures that the distribution and coverage of examination content matches the instructional objectives and major content areas.

Construction Tips

- The response choices should be relatively brief, with the major content elements of the question included in the stem. The content can include graphs, images, clinical scenarios, research findings or other complex information that requires interpretation.
- Write each response option so that it matches the grammar of the stem.
- Equally distribute the position of the correct response across a series of questions. For example, the correct answer should not always be the third response option. A strategy to avoid such bias is to always order your response options alphabetically or numerically. Knowing this, the students cannot expect position bias.
- Do not use "all of the above" or "none of the above" as a response option.
- Avoid questions worded with negatives or double negatives.
- The correct and incorrect response options should be about the same length.
- Avoid the use of response options that are irrelevant or silly. This increases the likelihood of guessing the correct response.
- One MCQ can be viewed as a cluster of true/false questions, where one response choice is true and all of the others are false. When using true and false questions, the number of true and false questions should be roughly equal, and care should be used to construct questions of approximately the same length. A limitation of true and false questions is that for questions where the correct choice is false, you do not have assurance that the students in fact know the true answer. Another limitation of true and false questions is that they require statements that are absolutely true or absolutely false. These types of questions are best used for assessing factual recall.

Extended-Matching Questions

The extended-matching question format was developed to address some of the limitations of the MCQ format. The major advantage over MCQs is that the larger number of response options reduces the likelihood that the question will cue the student to the correct answer; students also are less likely to recognize the correct answer. In many ways, the strengths and limitations of extended-matching questions are similar to those of multiple-choice questions.

Extended matching questions are organized around themes, and include multiple response options, instructions and a series of stems. Here is an example:

Theme: Endocrine glands and hormones

Options   A. Luteinizing hormone   E. Estrogen   I. Norepinephrine
           B. Vasopressin   F. Insulin   J. Prolactin
           C. Calcitonin   G. Testosterone   K. Oxytocin
           D. Glucagon   H. Melatonin   L. Progesterone

Instructions For each statement below, select one hormone that best fits the description.

Stems   1. Secreted by the thyroid gland.
           2. Stimulates ovulation and corpus luteum formation.
           3. Lowers blood sugar.
           4. Secreted by pineal gland.

Strengths

- This question format can be used to construct an exam covering a wide range of content.
- This question format can be used to test knowledge recall as well as knowledge application.
- Scoring is highly reliable and objective, and like MCQs can easily be automated for efficiency.
- This question format is often used to test recall of factual information; there is less of a chance of students recognizing or guessing the right answer compared to MCQs. They can also be used to test problem-solving skills such as clinical diagnosis or patient management.

Limitations

- As with MCQs, time and practice are needed to write good questions that take advantage of the strengths of this format but do not cue the respondent.
- Similar to MCQs, these questions provide only minimal feedback to students to enhance their learning. Some examination software applications allow additional feedback either during or following the examination.

Reliability and Validity

- Like MCQs, this item format has high reliability because of the consistency of scoring over time or across examiners.
- The validity of an exam using extended matching questions is based on the representativeness of the test content compared to the instructional content. Like MCQs, questions derived from a test blueprint can assure a fair test in terms of content.

Construction Tips

- Extended matching questions are usually written around a theme. When the theme is based on a clinical scenario, research abstract or an image, the questions can require students to recall knowledge, interpret findings or suggest possible diagnoses.
- The response choices should be relatively brief, with the major content elements included in the questions.
- Avoid questions worded with negatives or double negatives.
- Avoid the use of response options that are irrelevant or silly.

There is an excellent resource for extended-matching questions available at no charge from the National Board of Medical Examiners website (www.nbme.org). Under publications, look for "Item Writing Manual: Constructing Written Test Questions for the Basic and Clinical Sciences" by Susan Case and David Swanson.

Essays and Modified Essay Questions

These types of questions are characterized by the requirement that the student constructs a response rather than choose a correct response from one or more options provided. Essay and modified essay questions provide an opportunity to assess student's ability to apply knowledge to solve problems, organize ideas or information, and synthesize information. A sample essay question might be,

You are treating Sandy, a 57 year old woman who was diagnosed six months ago with Stage 2 adenocarcinoma of the right lung. Until a few days ago, her pain has been well-controlled. You have reevaluated the pain control and decided to initiate treatment with sustained release oral morphine. Sandy's brother is coming to the next appointment; he has concerns that his sister will become addicted to the pain medication. What will you say to Sandy's brother?

Modified essay questions are an assessment format that addresses some of the limitations of the essay question. A modified essay question is made up of one or more short answer questions. The student is provided with basic science or clinical information and then asked to write brief responses to one or more questions. When a series of questions is presented, additional information about the original problem can be provided at each subsequent step, guiding the students through an analytical process.

David is a 26 year old computer programmer, who lives alone with his dog Max. He has come to your office complaining of a persistent cough.

1. What are three likely diagnoses?
   a.
   b.
   c.
2. List five specific questions that would help you distinguish among these possibilities.
   a.
   b.
   c.
   d.
   e.

David tells you that the cough started about 5 days ago, and that many people in his office have called in sick lately. He has felt feverish and had some chills yesterday evening. He has been coughing up a small amount of thick green sputum.

3. List two diagnostic tests appropriate for work-up of this case.
   a.
   b.

Strengths

- This question format can be used to test written communication skills.
- Essay questions can focus on content related to knowledge or attitudes.
- Essay questions are best used to assess depth of knowledge within a limited area of content.
- This question format is familiar to students, and fairly straightforward for faculty to construct.

- Essay and modified essay questions are well-suited for formative feedback, since students can be provided with a model answer to help them understand their performance and prepare for future assessments.
- Modified essay questions require less time to score than traditional essay questions. Because student responses tend to be shorter and more succinct, these types of questions are less subject to scoring bias and can provide broader content coverage, both of which increase the reliability and validity of the assessment. While essay questions can be used to assess higher levels of student cognitive ability, modified essay questions are ideal for testing knowledge recall that is not based on recognizing the correct answer as in MCQs.

Limitations

- Reliability is a major concern and there is a need to assure consistency of scoring over time and when multiple individuals are involved in scoring. Scoring of the written responses are more subject to general subjective biases of the scorer, often referred to as "halo effects." In practice halo effects occur when there is a possibility of giving some students the benefit of the doubt more often than other students while scoring written responses. An example might be students who are known to be strong performers, or students who have done well on other parts of the test might be given the benefit of the doubt more often compared to weaker performers. The possibility of halo effects is more likely when student identities are known to scorers or when a single scorer is used.
- More time is required for scoring these responses than other formats.
- Tests based on essay-type questions are more limited in their content coverage because of the length of time required for students to respond to the questions as well as the length of time required for scoring.
- Essay questions require at least minimal written communication skills, and if communication skills are not the focus of the assessment, a lack of communication skills might limit a student's ability to achieve a high score even if they know the content.

Reliability and Validity

- Reliability is a major concern with these types of questions. The individuals scoring written responses might need to make some inferences about what the respondent meant because of poor written communication skills including organization, grammar and vocabulary, or due to vague wording. The opportunity for inference tends to reduce reliability.
- Reliability can be increased by having a clear scoring scheme developed prior to grading the questions. One approach would be to create a model answer and then allocate points to specific features of the answer, such as mentioning specific key content, presentation of a logical argument, recognition of a counter-argument or

alternative explanations, or whatever else is appropriate to the question. When possible, all of the answers to one question should be scored at the same time, by the same person. If multiple people are scoring the exam, then each should grade all of the responses to a single question. Each essay question or set of modified essay questions should be graded independently of the other questions, and when possible the identity of the students should be unknown to the person grading the question to reduce the likelihood of bias.

- To create a test with high validity, it is important to make sure that the essay questions address important content as indicated by the course objectives and overall course plan. Having several content experts review the model answer to each question can strengthen the validity of the assessment. This is particularly true when the question asks students to integrate concepts from across several domains, which might not have been taught by the same instructor.

Construction Tips

- Write questions that outline a specific task for the students. Asking students to discuss a content area is not as clear or helpful as asking students to compare and contrast, describe, provide a justification or explain.
- To improve reliability and the sampling of course content, it is more effective to use a large number of modified essay questions requiring short answers than to use a more limited number of essay questions requiring long written answers.
- Prepare a model answer after constructing the test question. This helps to increase scoring consistency by assuring that the answer you expect is reasonable given the question, and clarifies how points are assigned to content and presentation of the answer.
- To reduce bias and improve consistency, score only one essay question or set of modified essay questions at a time, and if feasible have separate scorers for each essay question. When this is not possible, rescoring a small set of answers can help maintain consistency. The subset of rescored answers should be sampled from throughout the set of examinations to make sure that the application of the scoring criteria did not change over time.
- When possible, score the answers to the questions with the identity of the students anonymous to the scorer.
- When used for formative assessment, student learning can be enhanced by providing students with a model answer as well as feedback about common errors observed when scoring.

Short Answer Questions

Short answer questions require students to provide brief answers to questions. The responses usually require only one or two words or a brief phrase. Short answer questions are often presented as fill-in-the-blank questions.

1. A middle-aged financial planner presents with a several month history of stomach discomfort. He has found limited relief with over-the-counter antacids, although these are now less effective than before. His discomfort is aggravated by caffeine, alcohol and late night snacking. What is the likely differential diagnosis for this patient?

2. In planning the diagnostic work-up for this patient, list two tests you would definitely include to aid in your diagnosis.

Like essay questions, short answer questions require students to provide a response rather than choose (recognize) a response from list of possibilities provided. However, because short answer questions require briefer responses, more questions can be included within an exam, achieving greater content coverage than with essay questions.

Strengths

- High content coverage is possible.
- This question format has high reliability and validity.
- Faculty find it relatively easy to construct short answer questions.
- This question format is familiar to students.

Limitations

- These types of questions tend to focus on knowledge, and are used to test knowledge recall and comprehension rather than higher level abilities.
- Scored questions indicating the correct answers provide limited feedback to students to improve learning.
- Scoring cannot easily be automated: this question format requires more time to score than MCQs but less time than essay or modified essay questions.

Reliability and Validity

- Reliability can be achieved by writing questions that are clear to the student, as well as writing clear model answers to each question. The distribution of points for the responses should be clearly specified. While bias is less likely to apply to scoring short answer questions, the likelihood of halo effects can be minimized by the same procedures described for essay and modified essay questions.

- Using a blueprint to create short answer questions that representatively sample from the course objectives and content is important. As mentioned previously, having several content experts review the model answers can strengthen the validity of the assessment. This is particularly true when there might be multiple possible correct answers for a question.

Construction Tips

- Write questions that are clear and specific.
- Prepare the short answer questions and the model answers at the same time. Afterwards, reread the questions and answers again to assure that the expected answer is reasonable given the question.
- To reduce bias and improve consistency, score the all the answers to a single set of questions at the same time. Rescoring a small subset of answers can help maintain consistency throughout the scoring process.
- Score the answers to the questions with the identity of the students anonymous if possible.

Faculty Global Ratings

Faculty global ratings can be used to summarize impressions of overall performance within a defined situation such as a clinical encounter, or aggregated over time to represent typical behavior in key situations, such as a clinical rotation or small group setting. Global ratings are based on a number of key domains of performance or behavior, with a judgment of the extent to which desired performance was observed.

1. Rate the student's ability to obtain information about the presenting problem in this simulated clinical encounter.

   a. Obtained little or no information
   b. Obtained some information, but with major omissions or errors
   c. Satisfactory performance with most information obtained
   d. Very thorough exploration of patient's presenting problem

2. Rate the student's participation in your small group discussion section with regards to his/her ability to disagree with or question others without conveying disrespect.

   a. Never
   b. Seldom
   c. Usually
   d. Always

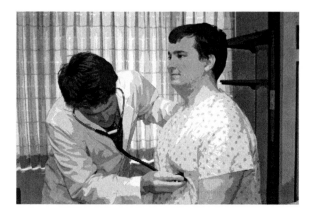

Strengths

- Global ratings by faculty tend to have high validity when they are based on the observation of behaviors of interest within a real or simulated context.
- This format can be used to assess general categories of performance such as clinical skills, problem-solving, teamwork, presentation skills and professionalism; participation and preparation in a small group learning context such as problem-based learning; or achievement of course objectives when used to rate group presentations.
- This format is useful in formative assessment to provide learner feedback.

Limitations

- Reliability can be variable when there are differences in expectations and standards among faculty providing the ratings.
- Faculty need to set aside time to observe students prior to completing the global ratings.
- Halo effects and other subjective biases are common.

Reliability and Validity

- Specific training to achieve consensus among faculty raters as to the rating categories and expectations for the ratings within a category is needed to achieve standardization. The rating form should have specific descriptions of the expected behaviors for each of the rating points within a category. To limit the impact of halo effects and other subjective biases, the use of multiple raters and multiple rating sessions is recommended.

- Validity is evident from the behaviors sampled on the rating form. Expert faculty can be used to determine those behaviors that represent the target performance in the learning context (e.g., PBL group, clerkship, etc.) where the form will be used.

Construction Tips

- The rating form should only include observable behaviors; these behaviors should occur at a frequency that makes them readily observable.
- Some people are better raters than others, depending on the rating task. Over time, it might be evident that some raters are more reliable than others. Using individuals who are reliable will improve the usefulness of the data obtained from the rating form for feedback and student performance decisions.
- The rating form should have specific descriptions of the expected behaviors for each of the rating points within a category.
- Halo effects and other subjective biases can be reduced through the use of multiple raters and multiple rating sessions.
- Student learning can be enhanced by providing students with copies of the rating forms to be used for assessment, indicating the categories of performance and the expected performance within each category.

Faculty Checklist Ratings

Global ratings as discussed above are frequently based on assigning scores on a multi-point rating scale for each of a variety of behaviors. In contrast, checklist ratings of direct observations are based on checklists that indicate the presence or absence of a specific behavior or a component of a behavior.

Please rate this student's performance of the following portions of the neurologic exam.

	Done correctly	Done incorrectly	Not done
1. Motor			
a. strength of arms	1	2	3
b. arms outstretched, eyes closed	1	2	3
c. strength of legs	1	2	3
2. Reflexes			
a. biceps (inside of elbow)	1	2	3
b. triceps (back of arm at elbow)	1	2	3
c. brachioradialis (wrist/forearm)	1	2	3
d. Patellar (knee)	1	2	3
e. Achilles (ankle)	1	2	3

Strengths

- Checklist ratings tend to have high validity because they are based on direct observation of specific behaviors of interest. The checklist represents a list of the specific skills expected of students.
- Checklist ratings can be used to assess specific skill sets such as clinical skills related to communication, history-taking, physical examination, or presentation skills related to a class project or clinical case.
- Checklist ratings provide specific feedback to learners about the elements of their performance judged to be present or absent.

Limitations

- Rater factors such as poor standardization, inconsistent expectations, and halo effects can reduce the reliability of the assessments.
- A limitation of rating forms is that for rating purposes, target skills are broken down into essential key elements. While this approach is appropriate and helpful for students learning a new skill, it is less appropriate for assessing the performance of more experienced students or practitioners.

Reliability and Validity

- Reliability can be improved by having clearly defined checklist items, and raters familiar with the skills to be rated. The less inference required of raters when completing the checklist, the greater the likelihood of reliable ratings. This also reduces the likelihood of halo effects.
- Validity is high for this approach because the rating forms are based on specific target behaviors, often broken down into key elements. For students learning new skills, this can provide feedback about specific components that were omitted or incorrectly executed. The items on the rating form can be based on the list of steps used to teach the skill.
- More advanced students and practitioners, with practice, will move beyond step-by-step performance of skills as they were initially learned to more integrated performance. More advanced learners are less likely to repeat the key elements in a rote fashion while still effectively performing the desired task. For this reason, when assessing the skills of advanced learners, global ratings might be more appropriate than checklists.

Construction Tips

- Reliability is improved when the number of options for each checklist item is limited. Frequently checklists are constructed with two or three options per item on the checklist, such as (1) done and (2) not done, or (1) satisfactory or

(2) unsatisfactory. Sometimes a third option might be included indicating that a step was attempted: (1) done correctly, (2) done incorrectly (3) not done. This format can be used when the student attempts a skill unsuccessfully, and there is reason to distinguish this from skills not attempted, such as when the rating form is used for formative feedback to students.
- If the checklist ratings are to be performed from memory, such as might occur when a standardized patient completes the checklist after a simulated encounter with a student, the number of total items on the checklist should be limited to what can reasonably be remembered by the rater.

Oral Examinations

An oral examination requires students to answer a series of preselected questions; these are typically based on standard stimulus information such as a patient case. Based on the patient information provided, the examiner can ask questions about differential diagnoses, pertinent missing data, additional testing, patient management as well as reasoning and interpretation of data underlying the student's responses. The length of time per case can vary depending on whether breadth or depth of understanding is desirable, as well as whether the exam is being used for formative or summative assessment.

David is a 26 year old computer programmer, who lives alone with his dog Max. He has come to your office complaining of a persistent cough.

1. List three diagnoses that you would include in your differential diagnosis.
2. List five specific questions that would help you distinguish among these possibilities.
3. List two diagnostic tests appropriate for work-up of this case.

   a. What is the rationale for each?

Strengths

- Oral exams can be used to assess knowledge and attitudes.
- This assessment format can be used to assess higher order clinical problem-solving such as application and synthesis of knowledge, ability to prioritize features of a patient case and evaluate treatment options.
- Oral exams provide insights into students' organizational and verbal skills.
- When used in formative settings, oral exams can be used to provide students with immediate feedback and provide instructors with information about students' approaches to problem-solving and reasoning.

Limitations

- Reliability can be problematic as a result of rater factors such as poor standardization, inconsistent expectations, and halo effects.
- Like essay exams, oral exams provide limited coverage of content and cases, which can limit the validity of the assessment.
- Oral exams require verbal and language skills, which can limit students' ability to communicate their content knowledge.
- This assessment format is not familiar to many students, which increases their anxiety.
- Time is required for scoring the results of an oral exam, particularly when a large number of examiners are involved.

Reliability and Validity

- Significant training of the examiners is required for reliability to be achieved. The training must address performance expectations and standards, as well as the use of structured rating forms to record student performance. The use of multiple examiners is recommended to reduce halo effects and other rater biases.
- Because oral examinations are limited in the amount of content that can be covered, longer exams are more valid than shorter exams. It is also important that the exam is standardized in terms of the content to be covered and the specific rating forms for scoring each examinee.

Construction Tips

- An effective strategy to improve reliability is the use of paired or tripled examiners for each question. Thus each student will have a different group of raters for each oral exam question. Each examiner should grade or rate the examinees independently.
- To improve the validity of this exam, the selection of the cases to be covered should focus on important content; longer exams are more valid than shorter exams because of the increase in content coverage.
- When cases are used as the stimulus for the oral exam, the same cases and questions should be used for all examinees to maintain standardization. However the order of questions can be varied across examinees.
- As with essay exams, model answers and explicit grading criteria for each question should be developed prior to the oral exam. All raters should be familiar with the grading criteria and rating form.

Standardized Patients and OSCEs

Standardized patients are actual patients or laypeople trained to portray a patient for teaching and/or assessment purposes. The standardized patient can provide a test of the student's skills related to communications, history-taking or physical examination. As the term suggests, standardized patients are used in assessment to provide a standard clinical encounter against which to judge student performance.

Standardized patients are typically used as part of an objective standardized clinical examination (OSCE). An OSCE provides an opportunity to assess student knowledge and skills that are not easily assessed using more traditional paper and pencil-based examinations. This assessment format involves students moving through a series of stations, with each station requiring specific tasks. Skills related to communications, history-taking, physical examination and written records are typically a part of an OSCE. A typical OSCE might be made up of about eight stations, each involving a 15-min encounter with a standardized patient, with 10 min afterwards to complete a written record or answer specific knowledge or interpretation questions about the case. In each of these situations, student performance is judged using the methods described above under checklists, rating forms, essay and oral exams. The Medical Council of Canada has used an OSCE as part of their licensure process for over ten years; an OSCE was introduced as part of the United States Medical Licensing Examination (USMLE) in 2004.

Strengths

- Simulated encounters provide a realistic yet safe context for assessing student performance of basic clinical skills as well as more integrated performance required in complex clinical encounters, such as deriving differential diagnoses, treatment planning and documenting clinical findings. The complexity of the encounters can be varied to accommodate the experience of the learners.
- Simulated encounters can provide students with immediate feedback about their performance. Alternatively they can be recorded for later review and critique. This review can involve students and faculty reviewing the recordings together, or can be completed by the student independently as a self-assessment.
- Simulated encounters can be customized to focus on educational goals and values important to the institution.

Limitations

- Despite the high fidelity of the approach, it does require some suspension of belief on the part of students.

- Simulated encounters are resource-intensive in terms of time, case development, raters and standardized patients.
- This format is unfamiliar to students and initially can cause anxiety, especially when used for summative assessment.

Reliability and Validity

- Reliability and validity increase with the length of the OSCE. Adding more cases or stations increases content coverage and improves validity. To accomplish this, the length of each station might be reduced to shorten the overall testing time per student. However, as the time per encounter decreases, the fidelity of the encounter might be reduced.
- In rating the performance of students during the encounters, checklists and global rating forms are frequently used. Each has their own strengths and limitations with regards to reliability and validity that must be addressed.

Construction Tips

- The formative use of simulated encounters is a very powerful technique and can provide students with tangible feedback to improve performance. In formative settings students often value this approach to assessment.
- The checklists to record student performance during a simulated encounter should be only as long as necessary. When completed from memory as is often the case when used by standardized patients, the value of long checklists and rating forms is limited by patients' ability to remember the specifics of the encounter.

Technology-Based Simulations

Technology-based simulations for performance assessment provide standardized conditions for studying and assessing clinical performance. Through the use of mannequins, computers, artificial limbs, virtual reality and other tools, simulations can be created for assessment purposes that provide a realistic challenge to students based on a clinical problem. The advantage of this format is that there is no danger to patients, and depending on how they are implemented the simulations can provide instant feedback. Written and computer-based simulations have been used to assess clinical reasoning, diagnostic plans and management. Simulators can be used alone or in conjunction with standardized patients. Additional information about this format is found in Chapter 7.

Strengths

- Technology-based simulations are particularly well-suited for assessing procedural skills, critical care decision-making and teamwork.
- When observed by faculty, this approach can be a powerful tool for improving instruction and providing feedback to students.
- This type of simulation provides important skill-focused training in a context that does not jeopardize patient safety.
- Technology-based simulations are useful for both formative and summative assessment.

Limitations

- Technology-based simulations are less realistic than standardized patient encounters, but can provide opportunities to demonstrate skills that might be impractical, uncomfortable or embarrassing for standardized patients.
- Simulator technology often is expensive.

Reliability and Validity

- Technology-based simulations create highly standardized test situations for students. Some simulators collect response data and provide quantitative feedback. This tends to be reliable and valid. To the extent that performance is judged on the basis of checklists or rating scales, these approaches each have strengths and weaknesses, which have previously been discussed.

Construction Tips

- A complete discussion of the effective use of simulators can be found in Chapter 7

Peer Assessments

Peer assessment is usually implemented based on global ratings forms; respondents are asked to rate the student's performance or to indicate the relative frequency of specific target behaviors of interest. Peer assessments are useful in that they provide feedback from multiple sources about an individual's performance, usually aggregated across a variety of situations or encounters.

For each of the attributes listed below, please rate the performance of this student compared to other students in the program this year.

	Well below average		Average		Well above average
1. Is professional in appearance	1	2	3	4	5
2. Reliable and responsible	1	2	3	4	5
3. Carries fair share of workload	1	2	3	4	5
4. Adheres to ethical behavior	1	2	3	4	5
5. Interacts appropriately with patients	1	2	3	4	5
6. Responds appropriately to advice	1	2	3	4	5

Strengths

- This format can be used to assess knowledge, skills and attitudes.
- Peer assessments can provide insights into professional behavior and teamwork, which are often difficult to assess using other methods.
- Peer assessments provide a credible source of performance information related to daily observable behaviors. This is especially useful for formative feedback when provided in a timely and confidential manner.
- Participation in peer assessments provides students with valuable experience in giving and receiving feedback. It also provides students with an opportunity to systematically compare their performance with the performance of others within a similar context.

Limitations

- Peer assessments can be provided through the use of rating checklists, global ratings or written narratives. Each of these methods has inherent limitations that have already been described.
- A general lack of familiarity with this approach is threatening to students.

- Some evaluators, especially peers, might be reluctant to provide negative feedback to their fellow students.
- Data collection, analysis and feedback can be cumbersome when used for assessing many individuals.
- A supportive learning environment is essential. When confidentiality and trust are not safeguarded, the validity of the data collected and the value of the feedback to students is significantly diminished. In the worst case scenario, peer assessments can be experienced by students as critical and hurtful.

Reliability and Validity

- A large number of respondents are required to obtain reliable ratings: nurses have been found to be reliable raters while patients and faculty are less reliable, which requires more ratings. This is particularly important when this approach is used for high stakes outcomes such as recertification. Individuals chosen to provide ratings should have multiple opportunities to observe the behavior of the student in question.
- Validity is a function of the process used to develop the rating form, the individuals from whom ratings are obtained, and the length of time over which raters have observed the target behaviors.

Construction Tips

- Students should know the rating categories used in the peer assessment in advance so the process is transparent and less threatening.
- It is helpful to provide guidelines and examples about giving feedback to others so that the feedback is constructive and appropriate for the expected level of performance.

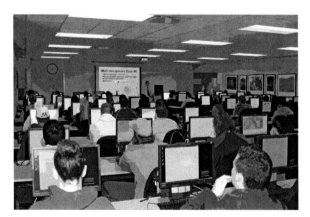

- The quality of the feedback will improve over time with practice; this is especially true for students, who frequently have little experience with this form of assessment.
- Peer assessments can be implemented as part of a 360 degree assessment, which involves ratings-based assessment of an individual's behavior. The ratings are completed by a wide range of others who have contact with the individual. In a clinical setting, this frequently includes peers, supervisors, instructors, nursing staff and allied health personnel; in some cases patients might be included.
- Peer assessment can focus on skills related to interpersonal and written communication, professionalism, teamwork and leadership.
- Although most frequently used in clinical settings to evaluate student performance, this type of assessment can be used in small group instruction, clinical skills training and other settings.

Self-Assessments

Self-assessment is often an informal process for students as they progress through their education. There are relatively few opportunities for students to use structured self-assessment for formative assessment; for a variety of reasons, some of which are obvious, the use of self-assessment for summative progress decisions is even rarer. The actual format of self-assessments can be written or based on rating forms, focusing on global attributes. Self-assessments are probably most valuable when used in conjunction with similar assessments from other sources such as peers or teachers.

Strengths

- Self-assessment provides students with a valuable opportunity to become more critical of their own performance as well as to develop insight and responsibility for their performance.
- Self-assessment provides a setting for reflection and creation of a self-initiated plan for personal and professional development.
- This approach can be used to self-assess strengths and limitations related to knowledge, clinical skills and personal attitudes.
- Because the assessment is self-generated, it provides a unique perspective on students' abilities, particularly when used with other information to provide formative feedback.
- The structure and content of the self-assessment form can be used to direct the scope of the self-assessment.

Limitations

- The most significant limitation of self-assessment is our own difficulty of seeing ourselves as others see us. This makes self-assessment a challenging task for many to do well, and even with experience, our inherent limitations in self-monitoring restrict the application of this approach.
- Since rating scales are typically the format used for self-assessment, the limitations associated with that technique apply to self-assessment.
- Students' lack of familiarity with a systematic approach to self-assessment makes this form of assessment threatening for many students.
- This approach is best used within the context of a supportive learning environment, where students feel safe to reveal their own limitations and confidentiality is assured.

Reliability and Validity

- Reliability can be increased by clearly specifying the self-assessment rating task in terms of the behaviors to be rated, the time period covered by the assessment, and well-defined criteria and standards to guide the assessment.
- The assessment should be structured using explicit criteria that are acknowledged and endorsed by students and faculty. This will enhance the validity of the self-assessment ratings.

Construction Tips

- The rating form used to guide student self-assessment should focus on specific behaviors and outcomes, e.g., what was tried and/or accomplished.
- To promote broad support and endorsement of the self-assessment rating scheme, open discussions involving students and faculty can be used to delineate the criteria for judging performance as well as elicit possible standards for each criterion related to satisfactory and unsatisfactory performance.
- This form of assessment can be combined with peer and faculty assessments to provide multisource feedback. This approach also helps balance unrealistic self-appraisals.

Portfolios

A portfolio is a collection of evidence organized around specific themes as a means of assessing knowledge skills and attitudes. The key components of a portfolio include a statement of purpose for the portfolio, examples of evidence selected by the student to document performance, as well as a reflective statement by the student regarding the portfolio content.

Strengths

- The task of selecting representative evidence of achievement provides an opportunity for reflection and self-appraisal.
- A wide range of evidence can be included in a portfolio including written documents and projects, letters of appreciation or recognition, presentations, digital media and resources, citations, logbooks of patient encounters, and survey results.
- The assembled evidence provides insight into the learner's ability to apply their knowledge and skills in integrative tasks, as well as the growth of their knowledge and abilities over time.
- A key component of most portfolios is a reflective essay that provides insight into higher level cognitive abilities as well as the learner's own ability to self-assess their achievements and what has been learned.
- Portfolios are frequently used for formative assessment, and can be an important source of information when combined with faculty mentorship.
- Portfolios can also be used for summative assessment such as faculty promotion decisions.

Limitations

- The task of selecting, organizing and interpreting the representative evidence of achievement is time consuming.
- Presumably the examples selected for inclusion in the portfolio are the best evidence the learner has of their performance, and therefore only a selective sample of performance is presented.
- This format is unfamiliar to many students and faculty, both in terms of putting a portfolio together and making judgments from a portfolio.

Reliability and Validity

- As with other forms of assessment, clear specification of the purpose and content of the portfolio is important to assure validity. The relationship of the portfolio to course objectives or promotion criteria enhances validity and helps define the types of evidence appropriate for inclusion, the number of examples to include, and the content of the reflective essay.

- Reliability is achieved through the use of multiple ratings of the portfolio content, as well as the use of multiple forms of evidence included in the portfolio to demonstrate specific educational outcomes or performance.
- Students and raters must understand the criteria by which the portfolio will be judged as well as the rating form that is derived from these criteria.
- Because the assessment of the portfolio is ultimately made through the use of rating forms, the issues associated with the reliability and validity of rating forms also have bearing here.

Construction Tips

- Providing learners with the responsibility to meaningfully choose the evidence to include in the portfolio enhances their ownership of the portfolio. Another way of promoting ownership is involving students in the discussion of how the portfolios will be evaluated: the criteria and standards to be used.
- Portfolios can include a wide range of evidence such as: an abstract or brief description of research or educational projects; publications or presentations; case studies; self- or peer- assessments; awards or letters of recognition/appreciation documenting professional achievements; conference proceedings or reviewer lists indicating contributions to professional organizations; awards; materials from websites or digital media that have been developed; personal reflections on specific achievements, activities, ethical dilemmas, challenging patients, etc. Almost any type of evidence might have value in a portfolio depending on its purpose.
- Software tools have been developed to assist in the compilation of evidence into an electronic portfolio. These tools range from blogs, wikis, online learning management systems to specific portfolio systems. See Chapter 9 for more information.
- Criteria for judging the content of a portfolio often focuses on the student's reflective essay regarding the achievements represented by the assembled evidence. The evidence can also be interpreted in terms of the breadth and depth of content, comparison of different types of content; areas of strength, weakness or achievement not represented within the portfolio. Another use of the portfolio is as a stimulus for discussion between students and instructors or mentors.
- An assessment derived from a portfolio can focus on the skills, knowledge or attitudes in judgments of the technical achievements represented by the evidence, as well as the application of theory or the ethics and values inherent in the content.
- There are circumstances when standard criteria for assessing portfolios might not be desirable, such as when the portfolio is implemented as a means of documenting the achievements and progress made by individuals as part of an individualized educational plan for independent study or remediation.

Reporting and Feedback

Feedback to Students

As mentioned earlier in this chapter, an important consequence of assessment is that students receive feedback about their learning. Many of the assessment methods described in this chapter will be used for summative assessment, providing reliable and valid information from which student progress decisions can be made. Some of these assessments are also well-suited for providing students with detailed information about their strengths as well as areas for improvement. It is this level of detail in the feedback to students that provides them with the greatest opportunities for learning from their assessment experiences and building confidence in their abilities. Formative feedback is also important for building confidence and reducing anxiety when students are confronted with forms of assessment that are unfamiliar to them.

Depending on the assessment, feedback can take the form of detailed model performance such as model answers for essay and oral exams, videos of expected skill performance, sample portfolios and the like. Other forms of feedback include summaries of the most common errors made by students during an assessment, and information about why a specific response choice was right or wrong. Of course, written comments related to the students' specific responses are very helpful but can be very time consuming. Another strategy is to have students self-assess their performance as a means of comparison with instructor feedback. To optimize the value of assessments as feedback experience for students:

- use clear criteria for grading performance
- provide feedback in a timely manner
- include both positive and negative feedback when practical
- make feedback as specific as possible

Feedback to Faculty

It is important that aggregated student performance information be available to the medical school committees responsible for oversight of the curriculum. Aggregate performance information can be used to provide evidence of the success of new programs, curricula or modes of instruction. Another important use of aggregated student performance data is to provide valid evidence for decision-making and supplement the perceptions of students or faculty. It provides a systematic approach to data collection that can be used to answer specific questions about effectiveness and outcomes, and perhaps give rise to further questions about the curriculum. Such evidence can be crucial in the face of personal testimonials or opinions derived from one person's experience with a specific student. This information can be part of an on-going effort to monitor an educational program or diagnose curricular problems as part of a systematic program review. See Chapter 12 for more information.

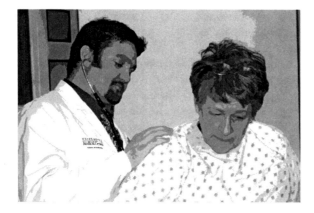

References

Case S, Swanson D, Constructing written test questions for the basic and clinical sciences. National Board of Medical Examiners. Available via www.nbme.org. This document can be downloaded free-of-charge from the website. Under publications, look for "Item Writing Manual."

A helpful resource is Cashin's paper, Improving essay tests. Available via: http://www.theideacenter.org/sites/default/files/Idea_Paper_17.pdf

For Further Reading

Amin Z, Seng CY, Eng KH (2006) Practical guide to medical student assessment. World Scientific Publishing Company, Singapore.

Anderson L, Krathwohl D, (Eds.) (2001) A taxonomy for learning, teaching, and assessing: A revision of Bloom's taxonomy of educational objectives. Longman, New York.

Challis M (1999) AMEE medical education guide no. 11 (revised): Portfolio-based learning and assessment in medical education. Medical Teacher 21: 370–386.

Epstein R, Hundert E (2002) Defining and assessing professional competence. Journal of American Medical Association 287(2): 226–235.

Fitzgerald J, White C, Gruppen L (2003) A longitudinal study of self-assessment accuracy. Medical Education 37(7): 645–649.

Gray J (1996) Global rating scales in residency education. Academic Medicine 71: S55–S63.

Hardin R, Gleeson F (1979) Assessment of medical competence using an objective structured clinical examination (OSCE). Medical Education 13(1): 41–54.

Holmboe E, Hawkins R, Huot S (2004) Effects of training in direct observation of medical residents' clinical competence: A randomized trial. Annals of Internal Medicine 140(11): 874–881.

Mancall EL, Bashook PG (eds) (1995) Assessing clinical reasoning: the oral examination and alternative methods. American Board of Medical Specialties, Evanston, IL.

Mehrens WA, Lehmann IJ (1991) Measurement and evaluation in education and psychology, 4th edn. Holt, Rinehart and Winston, Fort Worth, TX.

Miller AH, Imrie BW, Cox K (1998) Student assessment in higher education. In: A handbook for assessing performance, Kogan Page, London.

Miller G (1990) The assessment of clinical skills/competence/performance. Academic Medicine 65(9): S63–S67.

Raksha J, Ling F, Jaeger J (2004) Assessment of a 360-degree instrument to evaluate residents' competency in interpersonal and communication skills. Academic Medicine 79(5): 458–463.

Shumway J, Harden R (2003) AMEE Guide No. 25: The assessment of learning outcomes for the competent and reflective physician. Medical Teacher 25(6): 569–584.

Rademaker J, ten Cate T, Bar P (2005) Progress testing with short answer questions. Medical Teacher 27(7): 578–582.

Tekian A, McGuire C, McGaghie W (Eds.) (1999). Innovative simulations for assessing professional competence. University of Illinois Press, Chicago, IL.

Wallace P (2007) Coaching standardized patients. Springer, New York.

Chapter 12
Documenting the Trajectory of Your Teaching

Nicole K. Roberts

Being a teacher in a medical school is a challenge. It's a delightful, rewarding, surprising, engaging, inspiring honor of a challenge, but a challenge nonetheless. Whether you give lectures to large groups, facilitate small groups, guide teams in Team-Based Learning, or teach in clinical rounds, you are likely to find that as you try things out, you learn more and more about what does and does not work. The changes you make, for better or worse, plot the trajectory of your teaching – the ascent of a successful lecture, the descent of a difficult tutor group, the subsequent correction in style or approach that demonstrates your reflection on feedback or evaluation. Chapter 13 encourages you to be deliberate and evidence-based in your approach to improving your teaching. In this chapter, we will encourage you to document the trajectory of your teaching, and will discuss mechanisms for gathering information about your teaching from various sources.

Why go through the trouble of collecting information about your teaching, or considering how you have changed over the years? There are several reasons. First, there is the satisfaction derived from observing your own growth and learning. Documentation can facilitate your ability to reflect on your practice and to be deliberate in the changes you make.

External forces may also weigh on your decision to document your progress. For instance, with increasing frequency the public questions the cost, and the cost-effectiveness of higher education. Universities document their value, and within universities, individuals document their effectiveness in delivering on the mission of the university. For the teaching professor, this means not just being effective at research and service, but also being effective in teaching. In fact, in some institutions, promotion and tenure decisions rest on documented effectiveness of teaching.

What follows is a discussion of one mechanism for documenting the effectiveness of your teaching, along with some thoughts about materials that might be included in your documentation. In this chapter, we will discuss the concept of the

N.K. Roberts (✉)
Southern Illinois University School of Medicine, Springfield, IL, USA

W.B. Jeffries, K.N. Huggett (eds.), *An Introduction to Medical Teaching*,
DOI 10.1007/978-90-481-3641-4_12, © Springer Science+Business Media B.V. 2010

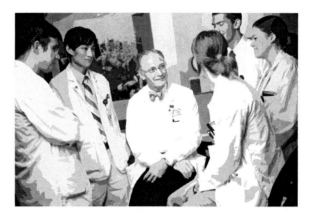

teaching portfolio, including potential content, uses, and structure. Then our attention will focus more on some specific approaches to gathering information that will be useful to the documentation of the trajectory of your teaching.

Portfolios

A portfolio is simply a mechanism to help you tell the story of your teaching to yourself and to others. It is a collection of materials, either paper or digital, that documents various aspects of your work as an educator. A portfolio can be used to demonstrate your effectiveness, show your growth over time, explain how you respond to feedback and evaluation, document your commitment to the teaching mission of your institution, and help you advocate for your promotion and/or tenure. Creating and maintaining an educational portfolio gives you cause to reflect on and refine your practice in a systematic fashion. It is also a method of communicating with others. You will likely share at least some aspects your portfolio with a variety of audiences, including your supervisor, a trusted mentor, or a promotion and tenure committee.

Essential elements to the educator's portfolio include the following:

Educational philosophy statement: Your statement of your educational philosophy will likely change as you gain experience and knowledge of educational theory. However, it is useful to think about what matters to you as an educator. What do you think the educator's role is in student learning? The role of students? How do you make decisions about what to teach, and how to teach? It will be useful for you to revisit your educational philosophy periodically to see how experience has changed your assumptions.

Five-year goals as an educator: As with your educational philosophy, you may find that experience causes you to change your five year goals; however, creating the goal statement allows you to begin to solidify what you want to do as an educator. It also gives you a prism through which you can evaluate new opportunities and make rational decisions about whether or not to take them on.

Educational contributions in any or all of five activity categories

1. Teaching
2. Learner Assessment
3. Curriculum Development
4. Mentoring and Advising
5. Educational Leadership and Administration (Baldwin et al., 2008).

Simpson and colleagues suggest the Q^2 Engage standard for documenting any of these activities: Quantity, Quality, and Engagement with the educational community. To document quantity, you will collect information about the types and frequencies of education activities in which you engage. To document quality, you will collect information about the effectiveness and excellence of your educational activities. To demonstrate engagement with the educational community, you will collect evidence that your work was informed by what is known in the field of education, and that over time, you have contributed to the field. Of course, your documentation will also include a description of the activity and your role in it (Simpson et al., 2007).

When you first document your educational contributions, you will likely collect all evidence of any of the categories listed. As you become more experienced, you will begin to evaluate materials, choosing those that do the best job of telling the story you intend to tell about your teaching.

For instance, you may wish to tell a story about how you are exceptionally responsive to learner's needs. To tell that story, you might begin with refining your educational philosophy to show why you value responsiveness to learner needs. In your philosophy, you might reflect on what in the educational literature suggests that responsiveness is useful and effective. Then you might review the instances of your teaching that were exceptionally effective in demonstrating your responsiveness to learner needs, and how you used a scholarly approach to developing your approaches to teaching – and so on for any of the other categories in which you made an educational contribution. As you continue your portfolio development, you'll want to continue to refer also to Chapter 13.

For help structuring a portfolio, you can download a template created by the Educational Scholars Program of the Academic Pediatrics Association. This template provides a structure and some concrete guidance on how to construct your portfolio, and it can be adapted to suit your particular needs. The template is located at http://www.ambpeds.org/education/educator_portfolio_template.cfm

Evaluation of Teaching

Some the key elements of your portfolio will derive from evaluations of your teaching and evaluations of student learning. In this segment, we will discuss elements of evaluation, definitions and purposes of evaluative activities, how you might go

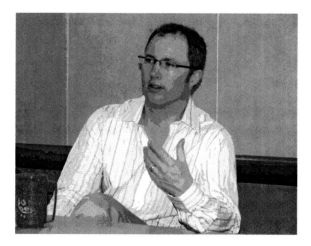

about gathering evaluative material, and what you might do with the material once you've gathered it.

Definitions and Purposes of Evaluative Activities

Evaluative activities span a continuum, from feedback to formal summative evaluation. Here we will discuss each of these ways of gathering information about performance. In addition, we will define some important concepts related to evaluation.

Feedback is a source of formative information. It is the first source of information you might seek about your educational activities. Feedback can be formal or informal, but regardless, its purpose is to provide information about the successes or failures of a recent performance in order to improve subsequent performances.

Feedback might include information you infer from watching your learners. When they lean forward in their seats as you lecture, they are providing feedback that suggests that what you are saying is holding their interest. Conversely, when they put their heads down on their desks, they are giving you feedback that says you have lost the battle for their attention. When your audience thanks you, you infer they got what they wanted. Though this level of feedback may tell you *that* something is going well or poorly, it doesn't give you information about *why*. For information about what worked, what didn't, and why, you should be deliberate in seeking feedback.

You can request feedback from various sources. Logical sources include participants in your educational activity, a trusted mentor or colleague, or even a supervisor. If your school has a teaching academy, you could ask a member of the academy to observe you. You might ask somebody in advance to observe your educational activity and tell you how it went. You could ask them to observe for a particular element or portion to see if it was successful or not. You could ask for a simple description of your teaching. Or you might ask to be videotaped and to have an expert review your tape with you.

In order to assess whether or not your teaching encounter has served its purpose, you might ask participants to tell you (verbally or in writing) what they learned from the encounter, or what they are still unclear about, or what they wanted to learn but didn't.

It's important to understand, though, that the purpose of feedback is to guide your future performance. It is not to make a judgment about your quality as a teacher. Instead, it is intended to help the trajectory of your teaching ability rise, and to make corrections when it falls off. It will be useful for you to keep a record of the feedback you receive and your responses to it, to demonstrate your willingness and ability to reflect on your teaching practice.

Formative evaluation. Like feedback, formative evaluation serves the purpose of helping you improve your educational efforts. It answers questions like "As of now, how are you doing, what is going well, and what should you try to improve?" It may be useful to think of formative evaluation as a mechanism to process and analyze feedback and to respond to it to ensure that your teaching continues to improve. Once again, there are several sources you might consult for formative evaluations. For instance, if you are teaching a formal class, you might distribute a questionnaire to your students in the middle of the semester asking them how the class is going. If your teaching is primarily in the clinical setting, you might ask your students mid-clerkship if they are getting what they want from the experience. You can use this information to adjust your teaching practices as needed.

Summative Evaluation. Summative evaluation is intended to provide a judgment about your teaching ability or your educational interventions. It is used to make a decision about a person or a program. Summative evaluations take place at the end of a given term, for instance, at the end of a semester or the end of a clerkship. If you are on a promotion or tenure granting track, your portfolio will be an important part of the information you gather to inform a very important summative evaluation, the decision whether to grant you promotion and/or tenure. Your summative evaluation should be based on a variety of observations from multiple sources.

Two important concepts govern the fairness of evaluations, and as the stakes rise in evaluation, each becomes more important. For quantitative evaluations, validity and reliability are important measures of the quality of the instrument. Validity is the extent to which the instrument measures what it purports to measure. Reliability is the degree to which the instrument reveals the same results on repeated administrations, or that multiple items within an instrument reveal similar results.

Levels of Outcomes Measured in Evaluation

Donald Kirkpatrick wrote the seminal work on evaluating training, and his levels of outcomes are often used in the education world. The four levels of outcomes for an educational intervention are listed from simplest to most complex to measure (Kirkpatrick, 1977):

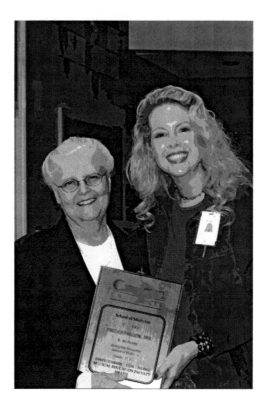

1. *Reaction*: How well did people like the educational intervention?
2. *Learning*: What principles, facts, techniques, and ideas did they gather in the educational intervention?
3. *Behavior*: What changes in their performance resulted from the educational intervention?
4. *Results*: What was the impact of the educational intervention on the rest of the system in which the participant works?

More recently, Belfield and colleagues adapted Kirkpatrick's levels of outcomes specifically for medical education. In their adaptation, the levels are listed from most complex to simplest (Belfield et al., 2001):

1. *Healthcare outcomes*: What measurable patient/population outcomes can be demonstrated to have been changed due to the educational intervention?
2. *Health professionals' behavior, performance, or practice*: What behaviors, performance, or practices can be demonstrated to have been addressed, changed, or implemented due to the educational intervention?
3. *Learning or knowledge*: What learning or new knowledge did participants acquire in the educational intervention?

4. *Reaction or satisfaction of participants*: How well did participants like the educational intervention?
5. *Participation or completion of the educational intervention*: To what extent did people complete the intervention, or how many people completed the intervention?

Kirkpatrick notes that not all levels of outcomes will be collected for all educational interventions, and this is true of the Belfield system as well. However, in the continuing medical education (CME) world, providers are expected to document the impact of the educational offerings at least at the level of showing behavior, performance, or practice change according to the new US Accreditation Council for Continuing Medical Education standards. If practicing physicians are the audience for your educational interventions and you intend to offer CME credit, you will likely be expected by the accredited provider to assist them in documenting the outcomes of the educational event at that level.

Various methods can be used to gather evaluative information. Below we present a table with the Kirkpatrick and Belfield evaluation schema and suggested sources of information (Table 12.1).

Table 12.1 Outcome levels and sources for information

Belfield	Kirkpatrick	Sources	Evidence
Participation or completion		Participants	Sign in sheets, roll call, attestation of participant
Reaction or satisfaction	Reaction	Participants, stakeholders, supervisors of participants	Written evaluation form, follow up polling of participants, follow-up requests from same audience, requests to repeat an event from a different audience, satisfaction of supervisors of audience members
Learning or knowledge	Learning	Participants, educators who receive participants at next level	Multiple choice examination, Audience Response System quiz at end of event, follow up survey of participants, survey of "upstream" educators
Health professionals' behavior, performance or practice	Behavior	Participants, coworkers of participants, supervisors of participants	Questionnaire for participants asking about behavior, performance or practice, direct observation, interviews with others who work with providers, interviews with supervisors, focus group with participants exploring behavior, performance or practice
Healthcare outcomes	Results		Quality improvement data from healthcare organization, public health data, prescribing data from associated insurance company

Summing Up

- A teaching portfolio is a useful mechanism to document your teaching trajectory
- Part of the portfolio is your reflection on your evolution as a teacher
- Part of the portfolio is documentation of your evolution as demonstrated by your response to feedback and evaluation
- Evaluation can serve multiple purposes, including guiding your growth and providing a judgment on you or your educational interventions
- Evaluation can serve to document the outcomes of your educational interventions
- There are multiple sources you can consult for information about your teaching

References

Baldwin CD, Gusic M, Chandran L (2008). The educator portfolio: a tool for career development. Faculty Vitae. Retrieved from http://www.aamc.org/members/facultydev/facultyvitae/winter08/leadership.htm

Belfield C, Thomas H, Bullock A, Eynon R, Wall D (2001) Measuring effectiveness for best evidence medical education: a discussion. Medical Teacher 23(2): 164–170.

Kirkpatrick DL (1977) Evaluation of training. In: Craig RL, & Bittel LR (Eds.), Training and development handbook, McGraw-Hill Book Company, New York, pp. 87–112.

Simpson D, Fincher RM, Hafler JP, Irby DM, Richards BF, Rosenfeld GC et al. (2007) Advancing educators and education by defining the components and evidence associated with educational scholarship. Medical Education 41(10): 1002–1009.

For Further Reading

Lewis KO, Baker RC (2007) The development of an electronic educational portfolio: An outline for medical education professionals. Teaching and Learning in Medicine 19(2): 139–147.

This provides a more detailed approach to developing an educational portfolio, and gives advice on how to create an electronic portfolio.

Hesketh EA, Bagnall, G., Buckley EG, Friedman, M., Goodall, E., Harden RM, Laidlaw JM, Leighton Beck I, McKinlay P, Newton R, Oughton R (2001). A framework for developing excellence as a clinical educator. Medical Education 35: 555–564

The framework developed in this article serves multiple purposes, but for somebody new to medical education, it can serve to outline the various activities that medical educators undertake.

Chapter 13
Teaching as Scholarship

Deborah Simpson and M. Brownell Anderson

Two medical teachers are leaving a meeting and a friendly colleague dialogue begins:

Dr. Charlton: "Are you going to the visiting professor workshop on effective teaching techniques tomorrow? It's the one about the relationship between adult learning principles and teaching strategies."

Dr. Cole: "I'm not sure. I really have to get my syllabus ready by early next week."

Dr. Charlton: "Oh, I can help you with that or you could contact the Office of Educational Services. I met with one of their educational consultants and in less than an hour we had updated and presented my syllabus in a way that she confirmed was educationally sound and she taught me how to upload it into our learning management system. If you did that, it would give you time to come with me to the teaching workshop!"

Dr. Cole: "You already get good teaching ratings. Why do you want to go to this session anyway?"

Dr. Charlton: "I do get pretty good teaching ratings, but I want to continue to improve. My students tell me that I have clear goals, I am organized, and they really learn a lot. I ask difficult and challenging questions, but in a way that is non-threatening. The problem for me is, I'm not sure what I actually do; I just teach. So I really want to understand more about what I'm doing that works and why it works. I've read some things by this visiting professor and his work is very informative even though it is not in my area."

Dr. Cole: Alright, you've convinced me to go work with Educational Services on my course and that I should go to the workshop. I'll see you there!"

Drawing inspiration, knowledge, support and challenges from our colleagues and from instructional consultants is how we enhance teaching and learning. Similar to the need to consult with colleagues about patient care or scientific investigators, we as educators must "get together" and discuss our work in medical education. Teaching, like any profession, "advances when people find like-minded colleagues

D. Simpson (✉)
Medical College of Wisconsin, Milwaukee, WI, USA

W.B. Jeffries, K.N. Huggett (eds.), *An Introduction to Medical Teaching*,
DOI 10.1007/978-90-481-3641-4_13, © Springer Science+Business Media B.V. 2010

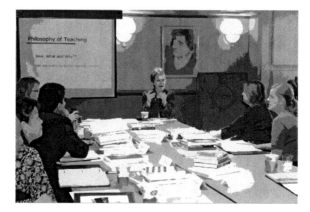

to work with, review their efforts and push them to the next stages of thinking" (Hutchings, 2004). Yet sometimes medical teachers work in isolation. We spend significant time and effort developing course materials, lectures, syllabi, assessment tools, standardized patient cases, and evaluation forms without first seeking existing materials or colleague review of our materials.

If you are reading this chapter, it is probably because you, like Drs. Charlton and Cole, are dedicated to educating healthcare professionals who will provide the highest quality of care possible for their patients, their communities and their populations. To achieve this shared goal, we as educators must think of ourselves as members of an educational cooperative – where we exchange and build our collective knowledge about medical education.

Enhancing Our Collective Knowledge About Medical Education: Adopting Educational Scholarship Criteria

Health professions educators should understand and adopt the criteria associated with educational scholarship as teachers, curriculum developers and authors of learner assessment tools. We should seek explanations for why something works or does not work. Glassick and colleagues (1997) have outlined six criteria that can guide our individual work as teachers and allow us to exchange and build our collective knowledge in health professions education.

- *Clear Goals:* The educational purpose/outcome is explicitly defined.
- *Adequate Preparation:* The teacher draws on the collective knowledge and resources in the field and has the required expertise.
- *Appropriate Methods:* The design selected including delivery strategies, tools, and approaches, is matched with the goals and best practices in the field.
- *Significant results:* Outcomes achieved are important to the educator and to the field.

- *Effective Presentation:* Educator's work is shared with the community, clearly articulated and framed to build upon the collective knowledge in the field.
- *Reflective Critique:* Critical self-appraisal resulting in the identification of strengths and opportunities for improvement.

Improving as an Individual

To improve as individual educators, we can use Glassick's criteria as question guideposts.

- What are our goals as educators?
- Are we adequately prepared for our various educational roles, be it as teacher, author of a curriculum, designer of an e-learning module, advisor/mentor, peer reviewer and/or educational leader/administrator?
- What are the appropriate methods to achieve our goal(s) in each role?
- How do we know if we have achieved significant results?
- Have we presented what we learned to our colleagues in an effective way?
- Have we stepped back and critically reflected to determine the key variables influencing our results and how to sustain and improve upon our success?

As educators we often seek to answer these scholarship-derived questions by ourselves. The "results" we review include student evaluations and student performance data as we seek to identify how we can improve. "Reflective critique" is informed by our experiences as teachers and as learners – as demonstrated by an outstanding teacher, a key role model, or mentor. However, at some point our ability to advance our own knowledge and skills as educators is limited by our own thinking, leading to the recognition that we are inadequately prepared! It is at that point when we must seek out other resources, drawing on the knowledge available in the field of education as a means to achieve our goals, expand our methods, perhaps reinforce our findings, and/or improve the effective presentation of our results.

Dr. Charlton is the perfect example of an educator who has recognized the need for adequate preparation. While students rate her teaching highly, Dr. Charlton is unable to explain why what she does as a teacher is valued by her students. Therefore Dr. Charlton seeks to enhance her preparation by drawing upon the collective knowledge in the field. Attendance at the workshop is an appropriate method to achieve her goals, but there are a variety of effective methods that draw upon the available knowledge base.

- Read books like this, reference materials, articles in journals on medical education and teaching.
- Talk to colleagues who are excellent teachers and ask them how they improve, what they would do in this situation, invite them to review materials and observe our teaching.

- Attend teaching workshops to learn how to write objectives, design assessment materials, and/or critique literature in the field.
- Critically reflect about a difficult teaching experience. This can range from an informal analysis to the more formal process of recording a critical incident and forcing oneself to step back and think about what worked, what didn't work and why. Share this with a colleague and get their feedback.
- Seek input from learners, asking them what worked, what didn't work and how to improve, both through informal mechanisms (e.g., at the end of a session), or through formal mechanisms (e.g., online questionnaires and surveys).
- Enroll in a faculty development program, medical education fellowship, or formal degree program to continue to build and expand your knowledge, skills and attitudes about medical education and opportunities and resources.
- Attend regional, national, and/or international meetings on medical education to learn about new strategies, techniques and resources in the field.

Replenishing and Enhancing Our Collective Knowledge About Health Professions Education

As an individual, Dr. Charlton can draw on the knowledge available in the field to achieve her teaching improvement goals. However, when we as medical educators only draw from the knowledge and resources in our cooperative community, we ultimately drain the reservoir of our collective knowledge. Our collective knowledge is like a river from which water is drawn to grow crops, when the water is not replenished, the river eventually runs dry.

In order to replenish and enrich our reservoir of knowledge about education, we as medical educators must actively contribute to our collective knowledge about what works, what doesn't work, and why. Again, Glassick's scholarship criteria can be used to determine the value of contributions to our collective knowledge. Does the contribution have clear goals? Was it prepared building on what we already know? Were appropriate methods utilized in its design, development, delivery, assessment, and/or evaluation? Were the results significant? Is the contribution effectively presented so that it can be understood and used by members of our cooperative community of educators? Does it include an assessment of strengths, weaknesses and opportunities?

To achieve the shared goal of preparing health professionals to provide the highest quality of care, as educators we must move from isolation (e.g., giving lectures, presentations, designing curriculum and assessment tools) to engagement with the educational community (drawing resources from and contributing to our collective knowledge). In 2006, the *Association of American Medical Colleges-Group on Educational Affairs* sponsored a consensus conference on educational scholarship. Building on over 15 years of work in defining the attributes of educational scholarship, the Q^2 Engage model emerged (Simpson et al., 2007). This model emphasized the need to transition from isolation as a teacher to engagement in a community

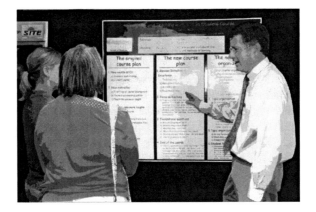

of educators. This engagement begins by drawing resources from and, as appropriate, contributing resources to the collected knowledge about how best to teach and assess our learners and evaluate our programs toward the goal of outstanding patient, community and population based healthcare.

Let's return to the examples of our two colleagues that began this chapter and use that conversation to highlight the concepts of how faculty can naturally engage with the community of medical educators consistent with Glassick's scholarship criteria.

Replenishing and Enhancing the Collective Knowledge Through Engagement

Dr. Charlton, who sought to understand *why* she is an effective teacher, did indeed attend the teaching workshop by the visiting professor, gaining a new understanding of how students learn. Armed with this new knowledge, Dr. Charlton then expanded her teaching strategies and skills, sought feedback from students and colleagues about her teaching, reflected on the results and revised her goals.

This continuous cycle, starting with Dr. Charlton's clear goal of teaching improvement, to adequate preparation via readings, workshop attendance, discussions with colleagues, through reflective critique demonstrates the use of Glassick's scholarship criteria. This process can also be used to guide an educator's stepwise development of instruction, a learner assessment tool, or a program evaluation instrument, beginning as always with a clear goal and adequate preparation by drawing on what is known in the field.

Contributing to Collective Knowledge Through Consultation and Presentations

For Dr. Charlton, her teaching successes resulted in several teaching awards both within her department and at the school-wide level. Over time, colleagues began asking Dr. Charlton for guidance about how to improve their teaching. She co-taught a local workshop sponsored by the Educational Services Office on effective teaching and was invited to serve as a visiting education professor in her specialty at another medical school.

During her visiting professor presentation, Dr. Charlton acknowledged the lack of significant results specific to effective teaching in her own specialty. On the way back from her visiting professorship, Dr. Charlton reflected on the audience's questions and realized that they highlighted the need for specialty-specific teaching effectiveness knowledge. Back at work, Dr. Charlton talked to several of her colleagues about this need with an emphasis on clear goals, adequate preparation as teachers, and appropriate teaching methods.

Inquiry into a Gap in Our Collective Knowledge

Through her *effective analysis* of the gaps in our understanding about specialty-specific effective teaching and the Q & A results from her visiting professor lectureship, Dr. Charlton engaged her specialty colleagues, her school's librarian and an Educational Services consultant to help her address this gap. The Educational Services consultant guided Dr. Charlton and the team through the selection of *appropriate methods* to yield the *results* that would answer their questions. The inquiry team then worked on how to *effectively present* and contribute the results to the broader educational community. Upon reflection, Dr. Charlton realized that contributing to the fund of knowledge in the field merely required engagement with her educator colleague community using the scholarship criteria in a stepwise progression beginning with clear goals.

Engaging with Your Colleagues to Address Gaps in Our Collective Knowledge

As practicing health professions teachers who seek excellence in education, questions and curiosities about the teaching and learning process emerge on a daily basis. Almost all the questions begin with "Why," "How" or "What." For example:

- Why did my small group work so well last month but not with this month's students?
- Why is the OSCE performance going up/down when we are teaching the same core content as last year?
- Why don't our students ever talk with patients and address health risk situations/behaviors (e.g., obesity, violence, smoking, unprotected sex, alcoholism/drug abuse – name your topic)?
- How can I improve my course?

- How can I get more students interested in caring for patients who are (geriatric, impoverished, abused) or who have chronic illnesses (diabetes, hypertension, asthma)?
- What would happen if I just stopped lecturing and put everything online?

As soon as you begin to explore your questions you are engaged with the educational community through reading the literature, talking with colleagues, attending workshops, and/or seeking consultations. By drawing on the knowledge in our field you can at least partially answer your questions and you will naturally begin to identify the gaps in what we know and consider ways to fill those gaps. Once you have effectively presented the results that fill a gap, you have contributed to our collective knowledge.

Table 13.1 Engagement with community of educators – Dr. Charlton's example

Focus of activity → Glassick's criteria ↓	Engagement with collective knowledge in our field	
	Individual – Draws From	Community of educators – Contributes To
Clear Goals	• Understand and improve own teaching effectiveness	• Improve others teaching effectiveness (colleague questions) • Answer question/gap in collective knowledge regarding specialty-specific teaching effectiveness
Adequate preparation	• Read literature • Talk with colleagues • Attend visiting professor workshop(s)	• Continue to learn about effective teaching (e.g., read) • Give informal guidance to colleagues in response to requests • Given presentations on effective teaching
Appropriate methods	• Try new teaching strategies/approaches • Ask for feedback from learners	• Listen to audience questions • Form a collaborative group with needed expertise to explore questions
Significant results	• Review results including student feedback, learning performance measures relative to goals	• Addresses a gap in collective knowledge related to specialty-specific teaching
Effective presentation	• Display your results in a form that is available for colleagues to review, critique and provide input	• Share those results in a form that others can understand and build from
Reflective critique	• Evaluate strengths/weaknesses and define specific goals for continued improvement	• Reflect on audience questions to identify gap → new goal based on recognition of gap in collective knowledge

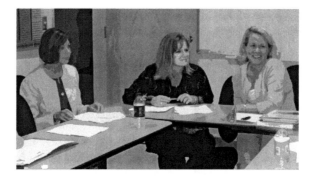

It is through this process of engagement – beginning with the question(s) that emerge through your daily work as a teacher and then drawing from and contributing to our collective knowledge about education – that medical educators can advance as individual teachers and advance the field of health professions education. Clear goals, adequate preparation, appropriate methods, significant results, effective presentation and reflective critique are the hallmarks of this engagement process (see Table 13.1).

Effectively Presenting Teaching as Scholarship: Adapting to Audience

What if this chapter had begun by advising you that your advancement and recognition as a teacher depends on your ability to identify an important question, design a study to answer that question, and publish the study results. Would that introduction have motivated you to "publish"? Would that introduction connect with your goals and motivations as a teacher? Effective teachers achieve their objectives by adapting their teaching approach to their learners' needs, goals and ambitions.

Our experience is that all teachers want to provide the best educational experiences they can for their learners so that their learners will, in turn provide the highest quality of health care possible for patients, communities and populations. However, when the emphasis is on "publishing" and "scholarship" the dynamic relationship between "teaching," "learning," and "scholarship" is often lost. Designing and delivering instruction, like medicine, must be an evidence-based performance art. To excel as teachers we must draw from the best practices and resources in our field and as professionals we understand the need to give back, adding to the collective knowledge in our field. Applying the Glassick criteria to our work as teachers provides a common framework making the relationship between our daily work as teachers and our contributions to the field transparent.

You May Well Be Asking, "How do I begin?" Start with

- *Clear goals:* What do you care about as a teacher? Do you have any "Why...,
  How..., What .... Questions"? Talk to a colleague to help you refine and clarify
  your goal.
- *Adequate preparation:* Read about it. Talk to colleagues. Attend a workshop or
  meeting on that topic. If you are interested in more information about teaching
  as scholarship, and how to document your work as a teacher, see the resources
  listed in For Further Reading.
- *Appropriate methodology:* Based on this preparation select an appropriate
  approach and try it.
- *Significant results:* Seek to determine if your approach worked! Engage your
  learners in this new approach by asking for their feedback and evaluation.
  Examine the data on your learners' performance, satisfaction and motivation.
  In addition to survey data, there are other indicators of effective teaching. For
  example, do your learners now arrive prepared? Are they early or on time (rather
  than late)? Do they remain active and alert throughout your session? If the performance data are the same but your learners report that your teaching strategy
  was more effective, is that a significant result?
- *Effective presentation:* Who else would be interested in what you have learned?
  Was this a question/problem of local interest only? You could address this by
  talking to your colleagues, holding a conference, sending a brief e-mail, and/or
  reporting at a faculty meeting. If this was a "gap" in our collective knowledge in
  the field (e.g., the literature, peer reviewed educational repositories) then tell us
  about it in a way that we can understand, use, and build on! As teachers effective
  presentation should be our strength as we constantly adapt our teaching to effectively communicate with different learners. Presenting our work to colleagues is
  merely another form of adapting to your learners!
- *Reflective critique:* Self assessment is a critical skill and one that is often hidden
  in our curriculum. Use the knowledge gained through your adequate preparation,
  selection of methods, results, and presentation to identify what worked, what did
  not work and next steps. And as you might guess this step provides you with
  "clear goals" for your continued teaching, learning, scholarship and engagement
  with other educators.

Reprise

To demonstrate this dynamic relationship let us pay a return visit, several years later,
to Drs. Charlton and Cole:

Dr. Cole: "Dr. Charlton, congratulations on your election as president of our Society
of Teaching Scholars! Your leadership will help us build new forums and expand on
our established sessions for bringing educators together to critically discuss how our
students' learn and how we teach."

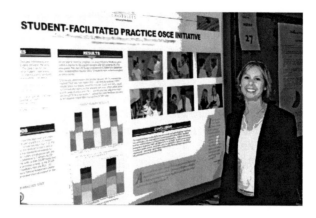

Dr. Charlton: "Thank you, it is certainly an honor. And I am glad to see you active in our society as well. I hope I can count on you to lead some of our sessions. I remember a couple of years ago when I had to convince you to go to our visiting medical education professor session."

Dr. Cole: "Indeed, your encouragement and nudging got me out of my office to work with others on education. I had always felt like I had to do it myself or I was somehow not fulfilling my roles and responsibilities as a teacher. Talking and learning from other educators has really improved my teaching and I even have some instructional materials on the assessment and management of common speech pathologies published in one of the peer reviewed repositories."

Dr. Charlton: "That's fabulous, congratulations! It often just takes some encouragement from our colleagues to prompt us to participate in the process of drawing from and contributing to our educational community. So can I encourage you again? Would you lead our education journal club for the next year?"

Dr. Cole: I'd be delighted to serve as the education journal club convener. In fact I was thinking that we might want to start an "Educator Reading Club" for our students and residents.

Dr. Charlton: "What a great idea! Are there some students or residents who could help you convene the group?"

Dr. Cole: "Yes indeed! One of my residents is a wonderful teacher and wants to learn more about teaching and learning. He would be ideal to help pull this group together... Ah, here he is now. Dr. Charlton, please let me introduce you to Dr. Matthew Scott. Dr. Scott is just finishing his first year of residency and is becoming a wonderful teacher. His students are always telling me about how Dr. Scott's golf analogies help them really understand..."

References

Glassick CE, Hubert MT, Maeroff GI (1997) Scholarship assessed: Evaluation of the professoriate. Jossey-Bass, San Francisco, CA.

Hutchings P (2004) Building a better conversation about learning. Carnegie Perspectives. The
    Carnegie Foundation for the Advancement of Teaching. Cited 15 September 2007 Available
    via http://www.carnegiefoundation.org/
Simpson D, Fincher RM, Hafler JP, Irby DM, Richards BF, Rosenfeld GC, Viggiano TR (2007)
    Advancing educators and education by defining the components and evidence associated with
    educational scholarship. Medical Education 41(10): 1002–1009.

For Further Reading

> Educational scholarship guides. AAMC MedEdPORTAL Cited 15 September
> 2007, available via http://services.aamc.org/jsp/mededportal/goLinkPage.
> do?link=scholarship

Four guides, each about two pages in length, present the key features of educational scholarship and explain why published educational works (e.g., curriculum materials, learner assessment tools, faculty development workshop guides) are comparable to other forms of scholarship.

> Hafler JP, Blanco MA, Fincher RME, Lovejoy RH, Morzinski JA (2005)
> Chapter 4: Educational scholarship. In: Fincher RME (Ed.) Guidebook
> for clerkship directors, 3rd edn. Alliance for Clinical Education. Cited 15
> September 2007, available via http://familymed.uthscsa.edu/ACE/chapter14.
> htm

Written for physicians who direct clinical clerkships/rotations for medical students, this easy to read chapter provides a brief historical perspective on educational scholarship and outlines it key elements with examples.

> Simpson D, Fincher RME, Hafler JP, Irby DM, Richards BF, Rosenfeld GC,
> Viggiano TR. Advancing educators and education: defining the components
> and evidence of educational scholarship. Summary Report and Findings
> from the AAMC Group on Educational Affairs Consensus Conference on
> Educational Scholarship. July 2007. Cited 15 September 2007, Available via
> "publications" link at http://www.AAMC.org.

This comprehensive report describes the conference design and format (so that others may build on the approach), provides the conceptual framework for scholarship as engagement, and provides a rich array of examples of how to "effectively present" evidence of one's excellence and engagement as an educator in each of 5 educator activity categories (teaching, curriculum development, advising/mentoring, educational administration and leadership, learner assessment).

> Shulman LS (1993) Teaching as community property: Putting an end to
> pedagogical solitude. Change 25(6): 6–7.

Shulman LS (2004) Teaching as community property – essays on higher education. The Carnegie Foundation for the Advancement of Teaching. Jossey-Bass, Inc, San Francisco, CA.

Lee Shulman, PhD is a landmark figure in higher education. He has held an array of leadership roles in higher education and began his career in medical education at Michigan State University and contributed to pioneering work in medical reasoning and clinical problem solving. Dr. Shulman is the Charles E. Ducommun Professor of Education Emeritus at Stanford University, and President Emeritus of the Carnegie Foundation for the Advancement of Teaching. As president, Dr. Shulman articulated, perhaps better than anyone else, the need to make what we do as educators' public, available for peer review, and accessible in a form that others can build upon, so that education becomes "community property." His writings are always a delightful read and should be an author whose work is on every educator's bookshelf. You can read additional essays that are guaranteed to promote reflection, clarity of goals, and remind all of us that we have an obligation as teachers to share and exchange our work.

Appendix
Additional Information About Medical Education

As your journey into medical education unfolds, you may want to refer to advanced resources in the field. Below we have compiled a list of medical education resources that should help your teaching career.

Medical Education Publications

Academic Medicine: This is the official journal of the Association of American Medical Colleges (AAMC). This journal publishes articles pertaining to the organization and operation of academic medical centers, emerging themes and contemporary issues and medical education research findings.

Advances in Health Sciences Education: *Advances in Health Sciences Education* is a forum for scholarly and state-of-the art research into all aspects of health sciences education. http://www.springerlink.com/content/102840/

British Medical Journal: The *British Medical Journal* publishes a series of articles entitled "ABC of Teaching and Learning in Medicine". The series covers various practical aspects of medical education. http://www.bmj.com

The Clinical Teacher: This is a publication of the Association for the Study of Medical Education. The editor describes the publication as aiming "to provide a digest of current research, practice and thinking in medical education presented in a readable, stimulating and practical style." http://www.theclinicalteacher.com.

Focus on Health Professional Education: This is a refereed journal sponsored by the Association for Health Professional Education. It is primarily directed at educators and students in Australia, New Zealand, South-East Asia and the Western Pacific Region. http://www.anzame.unsw.edu.au/journal/journal.htm

International Electronic Journal of Health Education: This journal is an open access online resource that is owned by the American Association of Health Education. The journal emphasizes international health education and promotion, and technology-based health education.

Journal of the American Medical Association: This journal publishes an annual issue devoted to articles on medical education. http://jama.ama-assn.org

Journal of the International Association of Medical Science Educators: *JIAMSE* is a peer-reviewed publication of the International Association of Medical Science

W.B. Jeffries, K.N. Huggett (eds.), *An Introduction to Medical Teaching*,
DOI 10.1007/978-90-481-3641-4, © Springer Science+Business Media B.V. 2010

Educators. This electronic journal publishes original research, reviews, editorials and opinion papers on medical education. http://www.jiamse.org

Journal of Interprofessional Care: This journal publishes original, peer reviewed papers of interest to those working on collaboration in education, practice and research between medicine, nursing, allied health, veterinary science and other health related fields.

Medical Education: This is published by the Association for the Study of Medical Education (ASME). Medical Education is a prominent journal in the field of education for health care professionals, and primarily publishes research related to undergraduate education, postgraduate training, continuing professional development and interprofessional education. http://www.mededuc.com

Medical Education Online: This is an online journal that publishes peer-reviewed investigations in medical education. http://www.med-ed-online.org

Medical Teacher: This journal is published by the Association for Medical Education in Europe (AMEE). Medical Teacher offers descriptions of new teaching methods, guidance on structuring courses and assessing achievement, and is a forum for communication between medical teachers and those involved in general education. http://www.medicalteacher.org

New England Journal of Medicine: This top clinical journal also publishes occasional articles devoted to the topic of medical education. http://content.nejm.org/

Teaching and Learning in Medicine: This is an international forum for scholarly research on medical teaching and assessment. The journal addresses practical issues and provides the analysis and empirical research needed to facilitate decision making about medical education. http://www.siumed.edu/tlm

Understanding Medical Education: This is a series of extended papers produced by ASME that addresses special topics in medical education.

Curriculum Resources and Respositories

Best Evidence in Medical Education (BEME): BEME is a group devoted to dissemination of information about the best practices in medical education. They produce useful systematic reviews that reflect the best evidence available for various topics. http://www.bemecollaboration.org.

Multimedia Educational Resource for Learning and Online Teaching (MERLOT): MERLOT is a free searchable collection of peer reviewed and selected online learning materials. This collection contains materials from all fields, but does feature a large repository of health sciences content. Resources are available for use under terms described by the author and users may also contribute content to the repository as well. http://www.merlot.org

MedEdPORTAL: MedEdPORTAL is a free publishing venue and dissemination portal sponsored by the Association of American Medical Colleges. It features peer reviewed online teaching and learning resources in medical education including tutorials, virtual patients, cases, lab manuals, assessment instruments, faculty development materials, etc. MedEdPORTAL covers undergraduate, graduate, and continuing medical education. Users can also contribute materials for peer review. http://www.aamc.org/mededportal

Health Education Assests Library (HEAL): HEAL is a digital library of peer reviewed multimedia teaching resources for the health sciences. HEAL provides access to tens of thousands of images, videoclips, animations, presentations, and audio files that support healthcare education. Users can contribute media files for inclusion into the library. http://www.healcentral.org

Organizations

In addition to publishing scholarly journals medical education organizations offer many other benefits, especially the opportunity to interact and network with medical teachers and scholars. The following organizations offer a variety of venues for faculty development and scholarship of teaching such as annual meetings, special conferences, online faculty development opportunities, etc.

Association for Medical Education in Europe (AMEE): The Association for Medical Education in Europe is a worldwide organization including teachers, researchers, administrators, curriculum developers, assessors and students in medicine and the healthcare professions. AMEE hosts an annual meeting and offers courses on teaching, assessment and research skills for teachers in the healthcare professions. http://www.amee.org

Association for the Study of Medical Education (ASME): ASME draws members from across the continuum of medical education – undergraduate, postgraduate and continuing. It serves as a forum for debate and exchange of information and promoting knowledge and expertise in medical education. http://www.asme.org.uk

Association of American Medical Colleges (AAMC): The AAMC is an organization of allopathic medical schools in the United States and Canada. The AAMC holds an annual meeting that deals with topics of interest to all aspects of medical education: organizational issues, research and best practices in medical education, student affairs and postgraduate training. The Group on Educational Affairs of the AAMC also hosts regional conferences devoted to curriculum and medical education research. http://www.aamc.org

ANZAME: The Association for Health Professional Education: ANZAME is an organization that promotes education in the health professions and fosters communication between educators in the health professions. AZAME's scope includes undergraduate and postgraduate training and continuing education. http://www.anzame.unsw.edu.au

International Association of Medical Science Educators (IAMSE): IAMSE follows the guiding principle that "all who teach the sciences fundamental to medical practice should have access to the most current information and skills needed to excel as educators." IAMSE sponsors an annual meeting as well as other conferences and faculty development activities and publishes a journal. http://iamse.org/

International Ottawa Conferences on Medical Education: This biennial conference is held alternately in North America and elsewhere in the world. This conference focuses on development of education in the healthcare professions by providing a forum for the discussion, debate and the reporting of innovations in the field of assessment. http://www.ottawaconference.org

Pan American Federation of Associations of Medical Schools (PAFAMS): PAFAMS is an academic, non-governmental organization whose mission is the promotion and advancement of medical education and the biomedical sciences in the Americas and the Caribbean.

World Federation for Medical Education (WFME): The WFME is a global organization representing six regional associations for medical education. It is primarily concerned with enhancement of the quality of medical education worldwide through establishment of standards. http://www2.sund.ku.dk/wfme/

Index

Breinigsville, PA USA
16 February 2011
255600BV00010B/188/P